COLLAGEN IS LIFE

COMPLETE GUIDE TO THE BENEFITS, POTENTIAL SIDE EFFECTS, AND WAYS TAKING COLLAGEN CAN KEEP YOU HEALTHY AND YOUTHFUL

DAN BANACHOWSKI

CONTENTS

INTRODUCTION

There are a lot of things that I could tell you about myself. For starters, my name is Dan. I am 33, and I am a sales engineer from downtown Chicago. One of my biggest passions in life is personal health. Every aspect of good personal health amazes me and fills me with ambition to strive to expand my knowledge and share it with others. Emphasizing good health and doing what I can to maintain the health of my mind and body is what I aim to do every day of my life.

One of my more recent obsessions with personal health has been working to delay the aging process–finding out what tricks can keep us as humans looking youthful far into our lifetime without all of the adverse side effects. Imagine my surprise when, one day as I was looking in the mirror to conduct my regular morning routine, I noticed my skin starting to show signs of aging. My deep desire to look and feel healthy drove me to try something that everyone touts as the number one solution to aging–botox.

Botox is known to remove wrinkles and smooth out aged skin. I went into the decision to get botox with excitement, brimming with expectation. I woke up the morning of my appointment thrilled and ready to turn over a new leaf; I was about to begin a newfound chapter of youth. After the appointment, though, I found myself not one bit impressed. It was not anything I had dreamed of, and the results were far from perfect. Disappointing, even. Deep unhappiness began to settle in, and it is a feeling I am sure you are familiar with.

I know what the aging process feels like first hand. In a world driven by pride in beauty, health, and youthfulness, it can be hard to feel good about yourself when you notice yourself starting to age. It can almost feel like a lost cause trying to delay the signs of aging–the wrinkles, discoloration, and more–and be tempting to just give up on your appearance altogether. Soon, you do not even want to look at yourself because you know you will be dissatisfied with what you find. Not to mention the fact that your health will begin to suffer too, resulting from the lack of motivation you feel to care for yourself.

As for me, I did not take that solution to heart. I refused to settle for anything less than the youthful, healthy look and lifestyle I deserve, and I was not going to hunt down some sham product that left me looking worse than ever with a lifetime of malicious side effects. After my experience with Botox, I started to do research on a different solution, and it changed my life. What I found was collagen.

Taking advantage of the benefits found in collagen has truly changed my life in undeniable ways. I enjoy dozens upon dozens of benefits from devoting time and energy to researching collagen and implementing it in my life. My body both looks and feels better than ever. As a matter of fact, collagen has been such a miracle that it cured a chronic ankle injury I sustained from years of sports. All of the lingering pain from the injury has completely dissipated after only two years of using collagen supplements. My hair, skin, and nails are entirely healthier than they used to be. The wrinkling I noticed has all but vanished and my skin has regained the levels of elasticity it lost years ago. I could go on and on about the benefits collagen has provided me with.

All of this is to say that I think you deserve to benefit from the use of collagen too. I want to make something clear–I am not selling you anything. Imagine a life where people admire your health and are inspired to work towards improving their own health because of you and your advice. You tell people your age and they look stunned, saying that you appear far younger and that there is no way you can be that age. Your bones and joints feel strong and healthy again, and you can do things you have not done in years because of the presence of chronic pain. I am going to teach you how to achieve all of these results and more because it is important to me that everyone knows how to take care of their body. Throughout the course of this book, you will learn valuable facts about what collagen is and how to use it to improve your overall health and increase your satisfaction with life. You are going to learn about all the options for collagen treatment, benefits, and any potential risks associated with collagen so that you can feel confident in the miracles it offers.

I know collagen as if it were the back of my hand now. I can genuinely say that I consider myself an expert on the subject. After years of research and consulting with dermatologists and doctors, there is not a single aspect of collagen I am not aware of. The benefits and drawbacks of taking collagen, as well as the exact science of how it works, are all important aspects of learning about the product for me. My passion for health and taking care of my body knows no bounds–I refuse to put anything into my body before I am sure of its results. With collagen, I am 100% positive that it is the product I need, and it is probably one that you need as well. I think it is not only important, but even vital, that I share all of this information with you so that the benefits are shared amongst everyone hoping to make a change in their health. You deserve to be an expert too.

So, without any further delay, the first step in becoming familiar with collagen and related products is to know what collagen is, how it is made, what the body does with it, and more about the biological science of collagen.

1

WHAT IS COLLAGEN?

C ollagen is a protein that occurs naturally in the body. It is actually one of the most abundant proteins your body possesses, making up around 30% of the proteins in your body (Collagen: What It Is, Types, Function & Benefits, 2022). The body is incredibly delicate, with even the slightest change in its composition striking the body and its systems as unsettling, dangerous, or even deadly. So, while slightly lower than average amounts of collagen will not necessarily result in something as severe as death, it is very likely if not assured that lower collagen levels will cause unwanted effects on the body.

Outside of just being the most abundant protein, collagen serves a very important role: It is the main material that the body uses to build muscles and tendons, skin, hair, and other parts of the body that rely on flexibility, elasticity, etc. Any connective tissues or parts of the body that have elasticity or bend often rely on collagen to be healthy, for instance. Science is not aware of all of the details regarding how collagen forms in the body as of yet–something typical for any bodily science–but what science does know is that eating well is necessary to allow your body to produce the appropriate levels of collagen. Still, though, people with even the most impeccable diet can experience poor collagen levels, which is because of the fact that diet is not the only factor influencing collagen stores in the body. Collagen is made, just like any protein in the body, of amino acids. In the case of collagen, the amino acids that provide it include proline, hydroxyproline, and glycine. In order to produce these chemicals, the body needs a plethora of essential vitamins and minerals, including (but of course not limited to) vitamin C and zinc, requiring further supplementation for some people.

The main processes that collagen is responsible for include growing and replacing skin cells, protecting your organs, providing skin elasticity, clotting blood, ensuring that bones and joints are connected by sturdy ligaments, etc. Specifically, collagen is responsible for:

- Improving and maintaining skin elasticity. In other words, it ensures that the elasticity of your skin does not dissolve and cause wrinkles. When you pull your skin outward and it bounces back into place, that is thanks to the power of elasticity.
- Replacing dead skin cells with new ones that allow you to appear more healthy and lively. If skin cells are not replaced, your skin can become dry, sag, or cause other more severe health issues.
- Strengthening connective tissues and joints. If you suffer from chronic joint pain, it is possible that you suffer from low collagen as well.
- Clotting blood, which means that collagen is necessary to stop bleeding if you are wounded.
- Providing a protective layer which surrounds your organs and protects them from various forms of damage. This helps ensure that slight injuries do not rapidly progress into more fatal ones.

Low levels of collagen are no joke; practically every part of your body suffers from this, from your head to your feet. And as unfortunate as it may be, low levels of collagen are not usually a result of the lifestyle that one chooses to follow. Instead, collagen typically lowers as you age, no matter what you do earlier in life. Things along the lines of alcohol, processed foods, etc., are not noted to have any spectacular effect on collagen one way or another, so while cutting down on these foods can help, it is not going to save you from the effects of genetics or aging on your collagen. You can definitely utilize foods and other natural sources of collagen to optimize your collagen levels despite this, but this is something that must be done actively and continuously instead of treated as a one-time preventative measure.

When taking collagen in the form of supplements, as many people including myself opt to do, there are a few important types of collagen that you should be familiar with. Each type of collagen serves a unique role in the body and is, therefore, necessary to make sure your mind and body survive and thrive throughout your lifetime.

TYPES OF COLLAGEN

There are dozens of types of collagen–slightly over two dozen to be exact (Llamas, 2022). It is not necessary to know everything about each of the 28 types of collagen, because in most supplements and for most people, there are five specific types of collagen that have the most benefits to reap. Those types are type I, II, III, V, and X, and I will explain what each one is and does so that you can make the most appropriate and knowledgeable decisions about the type of collagen to look for in your journey. These forms of collagen come in three main forms: Hydrolyzed collagen, undenatured collagen, and gelatin. We will discuss the forms collagen comes in more in a later chapter.

Collagen Type I

Type I collagen makes up the majority of the natural collagen found within your body. Accounting for approximately 90% of the collagen in your body, collagen is so vital that nearly every supplement on the market contains it. It is also the type of collagen that is perhaps most abundant in benefits and is very easy to source, making it a key element of most collagen supplements.

Usually, type I collagen that is not naturally found in the human body comes from cows or fish. This is because of the fact that both animals are already incredibly commonly utilized by human beings; we already benefit from cow and fish-related products via the food industry, so it makes sense that other parts of the animals' bodies would be used for collagen since they are already readily available. The collagen from cows is harvested from bones, lung tissue, joints, and tendons, which are the same places collagen benefits in humans (León-López et al., 2019). The degradation of type I collagen has been linked to many diseases, especially ones that impact bones and joints. As such, joint pains connected to collagen loss are often a result of the loss of type I collagen. All of these facts indicate that type I collagen is an important, hardworking form of collagen that is necessary to remain healthy and youthful!

Collagen Type II

Type II collagen is sourced from chicken and marine animals such as fish and other seafood. For example, chicken bones are a great source of collagen; therefore, so is chicken bone broth. As opposed to type I collagen, the research surrounding type II collagen is nowhere near as expansive. However, type II collagen has been linked to joint pains in the knees specifically and has been noted to reduce that pain significantly in combination with other over-the-counter treatment options (Llamas, 2022). Available research also suggests that type II collagen is easier for the body to absorb than other types and that it is beneficial in reducing inflammation and other joint-related ailments. The primary thing that separates type I collagen from type II collagen is that type I collagen impacts the bones and skin, whereas type II collagen is more joint-related. For those suffering from joint related issues, including anything from minor joint damage to severe disabilities like Ehlers-Danlos syndrome, type II collagen may be particularly effective in relieving at least some of the associated pain.

Collagen Type III

Type III collagen is the second most abundant form of collagen that forms in the body naturally, right behind type I. Similar to type I collagen, type III is also sourced primarily from bovines. This form of collagen is scientifically known to be best for bodily organs, including muscles, the stomach, blood vessels, the uterus, and more. The role of type III collagen is not precisely known when taken in supplement form, but the research available supports type III collagen as an aid for inflammatory issues. Little else is known specifically about collagen type III, except for the fact that those who have taken it noticed a myriad of long-term benefits from doing so.

Collagen Type V

Type V collagen is particularly interesting to me because it serves a far different purpose than the rest of the types listed in this section. Type V collagen is found in the human eye, and is responsible for our ability to be able to see light. Type V collagen relies on both types I and III in order to build up tissues in the body as well as to strengthen bones, muscles, and other parts of the body. It is simply incredible that collagen is responsible for such a vast array of bodily functions. From a scientific perspective, we understand natural collagen type V perfectly; however, science is not too sure about collagen type V found in supplements just yet. Type V collagen is super important to mention in my opinion, though, because of the fact that the research surrounding it is very promising—most of it suggests that collagen type V supplements are able to improve the function of the eyes, cells, and female reproductive organs. Therefore, supplements with type V collagen may just be perfect for those looking for eyesight-related benefits from their collagen journey.

Collagen Type X

For the last of the main five collagen types, we have type X collagen. Type X collagen, much like type II, is found mostly in the joints and is especially vital to bone development. Those with excess levels of type X collagen are more likely to have certain disorders impacting the bones and the cartilage, which is why it is important to take the right amounts of collagen to avoid potential health risks. This is something that I will explain in detail in a later chapter, so do not worry! The data surrounding collagen type X supplements suggests that it may be helpful to speed up recovery from bone-related breaks and injuries, though there is not immense scientific data to back this. However, science regarding the way cartilage supplements positively impact our bodies is at all times presenting us with increasingly optimistic advancements, so it is unsurprising that many people who take collagen type X supplements report pleasant findings.

REASONS FOR COLLAGEN LOSS

You now know where collagen comes from specifically and some of the functional roles it plays in the body, but what about how collagen loss occurs? Believe it or not, collagen loss is not something that just occurs from one central cause; there are six main reasons why collagen loss occurs. While most of these factors are not preventable and come down to biology or genetic reasoning, there are things you can do to naturally supplement your collagen if you are experiencing collagen loss (Miller, 2020). The six main reasons explaining collagen loss include genetics, stress, UV exposure, smoking, dietary choices, and aging.

Genetics

Genetics play a significant role in the collagen production of your body. This explains why certain people age "better" than others. If, as people in your family age, their skin tends to remain youthful and full of elasticity, chances are that your skin will be the same as you age. If your family is prone to wrinkles during the aging process, you likely are as well. Unfortunately, genetics are entirely out of our control. Nothing you can do will change your predisposed levels of collagen. This is the exact reason that you should maintain focus on other reasons for collagen loss, like diet and overall health, which are more easily able to be changed for the better at will. Even if you face genetic related collagen disparities, many of the ideas and tips throughout this book will be instrumental in saving your collagen levels and your health in the process.

Stress

Stress is another reason that many people experience loss of collagen. Stress is linked to inflammation in the body which causes the body to produce less collagen because of the rise in cortisol. When we experience stress, our cortisol levels rise, which in turn lowers our ability to produce the collagen we much need. Small amounts of stress are healthy, of course, but if you find yourself to be someone heavily stressed every day, it is a good idea to find ways to de-stress at the end of the day. Even if your skin looks and feels flawless now, that stress will catch up to you eventually. Maintaining a healthy level of stress will be good for you inside and out, and your cortisol levels will thank you for it.

UV Exposure

UV exposure can also cause collagen depletion in the body. If you do not already know, UV exposure refers to spending time in the sunlight. You might be thinking that sunlight is supposed to be good for you, but that cannot be true if it will deplete your collagen and make you age rapidly. That statement is not entirely accurate. Sunlight is wonderful for the body, as it provides us with a main source of vitamin D, which works in tandem with collagen to strengthen the bones and cells in your body. The danger of too much UV exposure when talking about collagen lies in not taking protective measures before going outside. The solution to collagen loss from UV exposure is as simple as finding a good sunscreen to wear before you go outside. Even on a cloudy day, sunscreen is vital in protecting your skin from the harmful UV rays we are subject to as a result of sunlight exposure. Ideally, the sunscreen you wear should have an SPF of 30 or higher in order to protect your skin the best. Any part of your skin that sunlight can reach, including your lips, should be treated with sunscreen daily. Not only will this help maintain the collagen stores found within your body, but it will prevent sunburns and cancerous cells from forming as a result of UV rays.

Smoking

Smoking is another easily preventable reason that collagen loss can occur. You probably know already that smoking is bad for you, but you might continue smoking anyway. Why should you stop smoking if you do not know *why* it is bad for you anyway? Alright, here is the reason you should stop smoking or avoid starting: it is one of the main preventable ways that collagen depletes in the body. Smoking replaces the oxygen your lungs should be inhaling with carbon monoxide, putting stress on the lungs. If the body has insufficient oxygen to provide to the cells, which happens to every single person who smokes, the cells begin to suffer. As a result, the body is forced to allocate oxygen cells to the most vital of organs first, like your heart and other organs, leaving things like collagen behind. Not only can the body then not produce enough collagen, but the lack of oxygen in the bloodstream causes cells to die, thus forming wrinkles as they do. If you are a smoker, doing your best to stop today will be a blessing for your future self, and of course, do not start smoking if you are considering it. You will be glad you did not once you hit old age.

Diet

The diet you maintain contributes significantly to how much collagen your body is able to produce. The number one type of diet that is damaging to collagen is any diet that causes inflammation in the body. This includes diets that make use of added sugars, processed meats and other foods, unhealthy forms of carbohydrates, and more. Foods like these are unnatural and bad for the body, triggering immune responses that cause inflammation and therefore reduce the amount of collagen production occurring in the body. Furthermore, sugar contributes to collage loss by hardening or breaking up collagen. As collagen works to provide elasticity, hardening it is obviously no good. This is why dietary considerations should at all times be made in such a way that considers the impact they will have on your overall health, including your collagen levels.

Age

Lastly, age is the sixth main cause for loss of collagen. Unfortunately, this is one of the causes that cannot be controlled–everyone ages regardless of if we like it or not. As you age, your body begins to naturally produce less collagen simply because of the fact that this is how the body works. Once you begin the process of aging, your body slows down on its production of various things, even if they are things we vitally need to survive. The process of collagen depletion begins in your teens or 20s, and steadily lowers the levels of collagen in your body from then on. Because age is not controllable, anti-aging tactics to support collagen levels are a must for anyone wanting to hold on to a vibrant and youthful appearance. While we cannot stop the aging process, we sure can work to slow it down or even reverse certain effects of it.

How to Improve Collagen Levels

There are, fortunately, a myriad of ways you can work to supplement the amount of collagen your body produces. Collagen supplements, which we will talk about more in depth later on, are a fantastic way to directly improve your collagen stores. Consistently taking the right collagen supplement for your body will stun you with all of the improvements it can have. Trust me, before I began researching collagen, I did not even know some of these improvements were possible! Now, I do not think I could live a life without collagen supplements knowing all of the good they do for my body.

Beyond that, the body also uses antioxidants to support collagen development. This can be found in oranges or other fruits with good levels of vitamin C, blueberries, and green tea. Because of this, it is essential that you keep what you put into your body in mind. It cannot hurt to throw some berries in with your breakfast or drink some raw orange juice every once and again, especially because of the fact that these nutrients benefit your whole body inside and out. It is also important that your lifestyle is one that supports good collagen growth–sunscreen and a healthy, balanced diet are necessary.

COLLAGEN MISCONCEPTIONS

Since collagen has become a hot topic in the media, and there is an insane amount of research and literature available on the subject, it can be hard to get tangled up in a web of misconceptions surrounding collagen and collagen supplements. In order to help you avoid these misconceptions, I will break down some of the most common misconceptions regarding collagen that I have heard and explain why they are untrue.

For example, the first misconception about collagen is that there is not actually anything you can do to restore collagen levels in your body once it has been depleted. Through diets, products like supplements and topical solutions, and lifestyle changes, you have the full power to restore the collagen amount and quality of collagen in your body. Because collagen production does not stop, just slows down as you age, it is possible to increase the rate at which collagen is produced when it is encouraged via supplements or other options. The idea that collagen is something entirely out of our control as humans is not actually as accurate as some people make it seem to be.

Another common misconception that people fall for is vague ingredients or additives that are introduced into products with the intent of selling a worse product at an upcharge. For instance, most marine collagen is, in fact, less effective than collagen that is clearly labeled with its original source. Failing to check the ingredients of your collagen supplement is one of the biggest ways to get tricked into purchasing something that you do not actually need or even want from a supplement.

Additionally, many people believe that the process of collagen absorption ends when you take the supplement, which is blatantly untrue and misleading. Just taking the supplement is not all you have to do; your body has to have the appropriate conditions for hydrolyzed collagen or collagen peptides to be transformed into usable collagen by the body. Collagen supplements you take are absorbed into the bloodstream via amino acids in your digestive system and other collagen peptides that already exist there. This action then distributes materials that the body needs to the rest of the body through the bloodstream as well, and then collagen can be turned into a usable substance by the body. It is important to know this because this allows you to understand that collagen needs a bit of assistance; through the diet and lifestyle changes that we will discuss later, you can help your collagen process in the body much easier.

Many people are also misconstrued in the idea that protein is an equivalent replacement for collagen. The same goes for amino acids. Taking protein and amino acids supplements as well as eating foods rich in both materials is a great way to assist your collagen's development and protection, but doing that is not exactly the same as taking a collagen supplement. In my opinion and from my experience, a combined approach of lifestyle and supplementation is best.

Furthermore, many people tend to think at first that collagen solely impacts their hair, skin, and nails, or just the joints. As you will come to learn throughout the course of this book, collagen is phenomenal for each and every part of the body, and believing that collagen only impacts a small portion of the body truly does restrict the potential that collagen can offer to benefit your life.

Knowing the various types of collagen and their purposes, as well as ways that collagen levels lower over time, is key to understanding how you can use collagen to your benefit for health and anti-aging benefits. Furthermore, breaking down the myths surrounding collagen is instrumental in your ability to begin understanding the benefits collagen can provide you with. Now that you know those things, you need to know what the benefits of taking collagen are in a higher degree of detail. That is where we will go next!

2

BENEFITS OF TAKING COLLAGEN

Collagen can be taken in many different ways and has dozens of benefits; some you likely do not know already about. It is actually mind blowing to find out about all of the different areas of the body contributed to by collagen. As one of the main building blocks of our bodies, collagen affects nearly every part of the body, both structurally and cosmetically. Before taking collagen supplements or dismissing them as unhelpful, it is worthwhile to know what all collagen supplements can do for you. I personally believe collagen supplements are not only miraculous but are lifesavers as well, and I want everyone to know just how vast and rich the possibilities are with collagen supplements.

For instance, collagen is a game changer when it comes to its anti-aging properties. Aging and corresponding signs of it are one of the main issues people hope to remedy when considering things like collagen. Most people view Botox as the solution to all of their problems, but collagen is way effective to a higher degree, far less risky and expensive, looks more natural in how it changes the appearance, and is guaranteed to give you results you will love. Without further ado, we are going to move on to talk about some of the benefits you can experience once you elevate your collagen levels back to normal.

SKIN IMPROVEMENT

Collagen improves skin in a few ways. First, collagen works to strengthen the skin cells, making them possess a higher ability to be resistant to damage or degradation. For example, when you go outside in the sun, UV rays can be responsible for the deterioration of your skin cells when you do not wear an adequate form of sun protection. When you have sufficient collagen levels, though, your body is able to keep those skin cells healthy and replace them as needed, like when you get a sunburn or dry skin. Increased collagen in the skin means that your skin is less susceptible to breaks and scarring as well as other signs of aging. When you get cut and the scar fades into nothingness, you have collagen to thank for that. On the other hand, if you have low levels of collagen, your skin is likely to be more susceptible to visible scarring. This also leads into the next benefit collagen has on the skin.

Second, collagen is known to improve elasticity in the skin. Every time you smile, frown, furrow your eyebrows, raise your eyes, or otherwise make obvious facial expressions, you stretch your skin out just a little. "Big deal," you may be saying, because you obviously have to move your face to function, but the effect that this minute amount of stretching has on the skin actually *is* a big deal. As you age, the frequency with which you have smiled or frowned, squinted or made an angry face, begins to show. This is why so many older people have smile lines, creases on the forehead, and other wrinkles on the face. Wrinkles also impact the hands, feet, arms, legs, and every single other part of the body because of the fact that all of your skin has been moved throughout your lifetime as you have grown, your weight has shifted, etc. With collagen, some of this elasticity is preserved and even regained, reducing the potential for wrinkles. As a matter of fact, many people who have engaged in studies where collagen supplements were taken noticed significant improvements in skin elasticity (Choi et al., 2019). This means that these individuals noticed wrinkles becoming minimized and even fading away entirely once they began collagen supplementation. Collagen supplements can have this effect on skin at any age, so even if you find wrinkles to already be a thing of contention, it is not too late. Incorporating collagen into your life can still show clear benefits.

Third, collagen impacts the ability of the skin to maintain hydration. Hydration, elasticity, and strength all go hand in hand to benefit your appearance. With better hydration of the skin, your skin maintains elasticity and will avoid becoming dry and flaky or colorless, which is definitely a plus. Collagen is able to absorb the moisture that your skin needs to have that desirable bounce and radiant appearance everyone craves, especially with age. Additionally, collagen supplements can also prompt the body to produce other important proteins that benefit your skin, such as elastic and fibrillin (Van de Walle, 2021).

Finally, there are some claims that collagen supplements can even prevent acne and easy skin conditions, but the evidence for these claims has not been backed scientifically as of yet. This may work topically by allowing cells to regrow in acne problem spots, by allowing dead or damaged cells to heal or be replaced, or to minimize acne scarring. Even if scientific studies have not backed this specific benefit extensively, trying collagen out for the other benefits cannot hurt–you might be surprised to notice your acne fading away. For more information regarding specific scientific trials involving the use of collagen as a way to reduce the appearance and symptoms of acne, check out the case studies section in Chapter 6 where I discuss a specific trial that improved acne.

The bottom line is that collagen has vast potential to offer for those looking to take it and their skin. From the youthful appearance to the healthy quality and texture of your skin, collagen has something beneficial to offer you.

Glowing Skin

Separate from strictly scientific results people enjoy from collagen supplements, there is also the fact that collagen makes skin appear to glow. Everyone loves vibrant, youthful, and glowing skin, which is something collagen can do. As opposed to hyaluronic acid and other chemicals people employ to improve skin, collagen supplements work fast and effectively to eliminate or even reverse damage from the skin, moisturize the cells of the skin, provide elasticity, heal wounds, and smooth the appearance of the skin. Do not get me wrong, hyaluronic acid is definitely essential to keeping the skin healthy, but collagen supplements can be a better topical and supplementary alternative for those with more sensitive skin types. All of these facets combine to allow collagen to gift users the beautiful, glowing appearance they at all times wish they had, even if they never even had that perfect skin before.

BONES AND JOINTS

Collagen also has the capacity to work its magic on bones and joints. One of the many responsibilities of collagen is to maintain the ability of cartilage to function. Cartilage is what protects your joints; it is a rubbery tissue found on every joint that, when deteriorated, can result in joint pain. It is between each and every joint in your body from your fingers to your toes. Throughout the long and complicated process of aging, your cartilage becomes weak and your collagen levels lower. This can make it painful to move certain joints, as many people who age experience. However, taking collagen supplements can improve joint pain and stiffness, as well as strengthen the surrounding muscles. This is because collagen works to restore connective tissues and cartilage. Those who experience degenerative joint conditions later in life have spoken incredibly highly of the benefits collagen supplements have had on their overall quality of life.

In addition, collagen supplements have proven them-selves beneficial to aging or injured athletes who have no plans of stopping their sport any time soon. Thanks to the power of collagen, many athletes including myself have been able to overcome severe injuries and lead a better life. Many sports injuries have to do with bones, joints, or muscles and related damage, and this is collagen's forte; with a collagen supplement, you may be able to resolve or reverse injuries sustained even years ago much like I did. This will allow you to get back on the field or to doing whatever it is you love without the pain you have experienced.

Your bones will also love the help they get from collagen supplements; these supplements are a great way to prevent bone breakage or loss. If you did not know, your bones are mostly made out of collagen. Bone mass lowers as you age just like collagen levels do, so taking a collagen supplement is benefitting the levels of both your collagen and your bone mass all at the same time. Bone mass matters because losing bone can lead to pain, fractures or breaks, reduction in strength, etc. Therefore, taking collagen supplements can help prevent such injuries alongside providing a host of other benefits, including nail and hair growth.

NAIL AND HAIR GROWTH

Collagen supplements have been noted to lead to quite impressive benefits for hair and nail growth. Just like your skin and joints, age is known to cause a significant reduction in the quality of your hair and nails. During the aging process, hair and nails can lose significant amounts of collagen resulting in breakages, brittle hair and nails, dry textures, peeling, and so many more unwanted effects regarding hair and nails. This is especially the case for those who suffer from a genetic predisposition to bad hair with age. Fortunately, collagen supplements are such miracle workers that taking them can counteract these nasty symptoms of age. With collagen, you are effectively strengthening the building blocks of your hair and nails and allowing them to successfully grow in a much healthier way. Just like your skin, dead or dying cells are healed and replaced which lets your hair shine and remain strong.

As far as nails go, collagen improves nail growth by strengthening your nails and providing them with much needed flexibility. You might be thinking that you do not want flexible nails, you want strong ones. And you are right; too much flexibility in the nails is definitely a bad thing. However, in the case of collagen, the supplement allows your nails to have just enough flexibility that if you hit your nails against something, for example, they bend enough to prevent breakage. Without that flexibility, your nails would break at many different types of minor pressure, and no one wants that. This is effectively what people refer to as "brittle nails." Sufficient collagen is also needed to allow your nails to grow smooth, hydrated, and healthy. To prevent your nails from breaking, peeling, chipping, cracking, or bending too much, collagen is the way to go.

These positive effects also extend to the hair. Your hair, skin, and nails often come in a combined package when it comes to health and supplements, so it makes sense that it is the same for collagen. Collagen provides two main benefits to the hair in order to stimulate growth and health: Amino acid production and protection in various forms (The Benefits of Collagen for Hair, Skin & Nails, 2020). It is essential for healthy hair to have various amino acids in order to grow. For example, one of the most important amino acids employed by the hair is keratin, which you may have heard of already, especially if you are a fan of hair care products. Keratin needs both essential and non-essential amino acids, and while the body can produce those essential amino acids, it cannot produce the non-essential ones. Non-essential amino acids are gained solely from the diet that someone chooses to follow, and collagen conveniently contains three different non-essential amino acids that allow keratin formation, thus leading to hair growth.

Who knew a simple supplement could pack so much power?

Collagen also provides protection to the hair itself, mainly from something that is called "oxidative stress." As mentioned earlier, collagen is an antioxidant and is furthermore reliant on the strength of antioxidants to supplement its own abilities. This means that collagen has the capacity to protect cells from something called free radicals, a reactive form of oxygen that can degrade the quality of hair, skin, and nails. Because collagen is an antioxidant that protects from free radicals, collagen supplements have the power to protect hair from thinning, graying, and loss associated with age. This means that if you are worried about your hair as you get older, collagen is the right way to go about protecting it.

HEART HEALTH

The list goes on! The next benefit you can enjoy as a result of collagen supplements is improved heart health (Turner, 2022). Collagen is good for the heart in many ways. First, collagen ensures that arteries remain in pristine condition. As you age, depending on your lifestyle and genetics, your arteries can become stiff or weak, preventing adequate blood flow from the heart to the rest of your body. Blood needs to be able to flow to every area of your body, yet as you age, that ability slowly starts to decline. Weak arteries can lead to increased risk of heart disease, heart attacks, and stroke. Collagen is able to provide arteries with the resources they need to remain flexible and strong as you age, making sure that blood flows everywhere it needs to go.

Collagen is also wonderful at keeping cholesterol to a healthy level. You may already know that high cholesterol levels can cause heart problems. This situation arises because cholesterol loves to form plaque inside of the arterial walls, making the pathways inside of your arteries far more narrow. Too much plaque inside of the arteries can lower blood flow or stop it altogether, increasing the risk of stroke and heart attack. Collagen supplements are able to decrease cholesterol levels as well as harmful fats in the body, keeping the arteries clear and in tip-top shape. You should, of course, be making adequate dietary choices to reduce your risk of high cholesterol and clogged arteries, but for those who are worried or have that dreaded genetic predisposition, I highly suggest collagen to soothe your worries.

Blood pressure is yet another facet of heart health that collagen can aid in improving. High blood pressure often is a result of what I mentioned before–the narrowing of arterial pathways due to plaque buildup. Glycine, an amino acid inside of collagen, is able to reduce blood pressure and protect the heart in this way too. Research also suggests that collagen is able to raise levels of nitric oxide, something responsible for regulating blood flow and blood pressure in the body. Because of the way collagen behaves in correlation with blood pressure and the heart, many people have reported significant improvements in mild hypertension as a result of taking collagen supplements regularly.

Finally, collagen helps maintain heart health by keeping your level of inflammation low. This is especially beneficial for people who have arthritis or are incredibly physically active on a regular basis. Collagen does this by preventing chemicals in the body that cause inflammatory responses from working, which might sound bad if you think about it and do not know much about inflammation, but truly, you do not want any inflammation in the body. Glycine found in collagen is well known to play a key role in reducing inflammation as well, and studies have shown that low levels of glycine can cause an increased risk of heart attacks. Using collagen to boost glycine levels in the body is a sure-fire way to care for your heart!

GUT HEALTH

Studies also show that collagen is useful for improving the health of your gut (Is Collagen Good for Gut Health?, n.d.). Gut health refers to a balance of bacteria in your throat, stomach, and intestine, all components of your digestive system, which allow for proper digestion of the food we eat. If there is not a proper balance between the bacteria in these locations, we suffer from digestive issues like bloating, stomachaches, constipation, etc. Everything you eat passess through the gut, which allows us to gain nutrients from our food as well as rid our bodies of waste. Maintaining good gut health allows you to be healthy and prevents various illnesses from flourishing in your body. Collagen is able to ensure gut health by repairing the lining of your digestive system with those powerful amino acids it carries, making sure that the stomach and associated components of digestion are healthy and in tip-top shape for balancing bacteria.

Glycine and proline, two compounds contained within collagen, are also incredibly beneficial for the health of your gut. Collagen works to repair the inside of your stomach and related parts of the body by building upon the tissue, which can prevent various forms of sickness including irritable bowel syndrome, or IBS. Incorporating a collagen supplement into your diet if you have stomach problems could potentially resolve a variety of the ailments you are facing, and it will protect the health of your gut as you age as well.

INJURY RECOVERY

I mentioned earlier that collagen supplements were life-changing for a chronic pain injury in my ankle that I sustained from years of sports. It is not at all shocking that collagen has the ability to do this. In fact, collagen has the power to reinforce many parts of the body that can be damaged during various points in engaging with sports, and can even go as far as healing existing injuries that otherwise might be permanent (5 Research Studies That Show That Collagen Protein Should Be a Part of Your Sports Injury Treatment, n.d.). Even if you are not an athlete or lead a relatively sedentary lifestyle, the benefits that collagen has on the body can be enjoyed universally by anyone who is prone to injury (and that is pretty much all of us) or has a family history of arthritis, Ehlers-Danlos syndrome, fibromyalgia, or any other incredibly painful chronic condition.

One way that collagen works to prevent and heal sports-related injuries is by improving the ability of muscles throughout the body to recover, which is an essential part of healing from any sports injury. The main benefit that people notice as a result of including a collagen supplement in their sports regime is less soreness in their muscles. As it turns out, collagen is an awesome way to speed up the process of healing from muscle soreness overall. Participants in studies regarding the impact of collagen on the muscles even noted that collagen decreased the amount of muscle soreness during and just after a workout as well. All of this is possible because of the way collagen acts as a building block for your muscles, joints, and anything else that can hurt as an end result of injury or illness.

Additionally, ankle injuries much like the one I suffered from are all too common within athletes, as anyone who plays sport knows well. Spraining, or otherwise injuring, an ankle is no joke. Once you lose stability in your ankle, it can impact your ability to do all sorts of things and can ultimately result in a permanent instability throughout the body. A messed up ankle has the potential to harm your knees, hips, and spine as well. Fortunately for us all, collagen has been observed in many double-blind studies to be great at improving ankle stability due to the properties it possesses. This makes collagen a must have for fans of sports, running, or even pleasant evening walks. Collagen rocks both as a treatment and a preventative measure for the stability of your ankles.

Your ankles are not the only joint that collagen can help you with the recovery of. Collagen is also amazing at allowing your knees to be strong enough to avoid injury, as well as speeding up the recovery process for any knee injuries you may sustain. Studies of athletes with severe knee pain relating to functional knee problems exhibited shocking levels of recovery; significant pain relief was enjoyed by all participants in the study who took the collagen supplements offered. If chronic knee pain is something that is plaguing you, especially as you get older, a collagen supplement could be exactly what you need. The strength and support it provides can alleviate most of, or all of, your pain depending on the cause and level of severity.

Furthermore, collagen has also proven itself to be stellar at hastening the process of wounds like scrapes or cuts. Even in older age when the body is far more hesitant to recover in a timely manner, collagen can rescue you from the slow, agonizing recovery process that you may feel resigned to. Collagen supplements for wounds will allow the skin to come back faster and stronger than ever, and will also help relieve some of the associated pain. Collagen gel has been proven to be significantly more than effective at healing wounds as a topical treatment as well, which I cover in depth as a part of the case studies section of this book. Turns out collagen application is great for the inside of your body as well as the outside.

And finally, to the surprise of many people unfamiliar with the range of benefits this substance can offer, collagen is an effective way to get through the frostbite recovery process much faster. Many people forget about the potential for frostbite when considering sports injuries or injuries in general, but frostbite is one of the most deadly and painful injuries you could possibly overlook. Even just living in a cold area puts you at risk for this deadly injury, and avoiding it at all costs is essential. Across various studies, collagen supplements have shown significant improvement in under 24 hours for patients experiencing even the most severe frostbite related injuries. Especially if you live somewhere cold or love winter sports like skiing, collagen can prove vital to your personal health.

ACNE

Despite what movies, pop culture, and TV may tell us, acne is something that can happen at any age–it is not just a problem for teenagers. Being an adult with acne can be embarrassing because of the fact that we live in a society so used to considering that to be an issue for youngsters. It can cause anxiety, low self-esteem, depression, and a range of other mental health issues to suffer from acne, even at any age. It can be especially frustrating to suffer from acne later in life because at that point, you probably feel like you have tried every scrub, cleanser, and cream on the market to put your acne at bay. Something you might not have considered to be a solution for acne is collagen.

Collagen makes up about 80% of your skin, so it is practically a given that a healthier amount of collagen will provide improvements in the health of your skin . This includes acne. The proline found in collagen is great at reducing inflammation and redness associated with acne, and the reduction in inflammation removes the environment that acne-causing bacteria love from your skin. Collagen is also very hydrating for the skin, which prevents bacteria, dryness, and oily skin as well. Some people even claim that collagen has helped relieve them of acne scarring in the form of hyperpigmentation and indentation. If you have suffered from unrelenting acne or acne-related issues throughout your whole life, it is possible that a little collagen is all you need to start developing the smooth, healthy skin of your dreams.

WEIGHT LOSS

If weight loss is among your personal health goals, it turns out that collagen has myriad benefits in store for you too. Collagen is effective at aiding in weight loss in more ways than one. Collagen has been proven incredibly beneficial for not just aiding in the process of losing weight but also in maintaining weight after it has been lost, making it a helpful supplement for anyone searching for an ideal dietary supplement. It is much safer than many dietary supplements on the market because collagen is well researched and lacks the gimmicky aspects of weight loss supplements advertised online.

One of the reasons that collagen works so well for weight loss is that it provides you with a sense of fullness from your food (Further Food, 2017). It is common knowledge that eating protein will fill you up, but collagen goes above and beyond in regard to that statement. Collagen studies showed that collagen tended to be 40% more filling than other proteins and also resulted in participants eating less at their next meal. Protein powders are a common tool used to satiate hunger or be filling throughout the day; however, these powders are often rife with fillers and flavoring that is not necessarily good for you. On the other hand, collagen being perfectly natural is great for the body and produces a similar satiating effect. Taking collagen as a means to provide fullness leads to a lowered tendency to overeat or eat out of boredom as well.

In addition, collagen has shown potential benefits regarding appetite suppression. Those studied in experiments tended to exhibit signs of a reduced appetite after introducing collagen into their diet, which was beneficial especially in the case of diabetic patients. Additionally, collagen is a protein and including high levels of collagen into your diet essentially incorporates a significantly larger amount of protein. Protein is a very filling nutrient, which is why it is typically recommended that you snack on proteins instead of sugars. The benefit of taking collagen for appetite suppression is that it subdues cravings and can deter binge eating, thus improving overall health.

I also discussed earlier how collagen is useful for building or improving muscle mass. This is also useful for weight loss, because it aids in the ability of your body to retain muscle mass during the weight loss process instead of losing the muscle mass you have in the process of weight loss. The benefits of using collagen to maintain muscle mass during weight loss extend so far; collagen also ensures that your body is able to stay active and that you will sustain less injuries during weight loss related exercise. Muscle mass development is also a good way to maintain weight if you are solely looking to lose fat content in the body without actually dropping your weight, which means that collagen can help you meet this goal easily.

Finally, collagen is beneficial for weight loss because of the fact that it can assist in preventing the occurrence or appearance of cellulite and similar visible signs of weight change. During the processes of aging and weight change alike, cellulite can appear and give the body a bumpy or unsatisfying appearance. Collagen supplements help strengthen the tissue responsible for visible cellulite, making it a must have tool for anyone undergoing weight loss. Beyond that, collagen can be helpful for reducing the appearance of stretch marks by strengthening the skin and returning some of the elasticity that was lost during the process of significant weight change. For anyone worried about visible signs of weight loss or gain, taking a collagen supplement will help you out drastically.

MUSCLE GROWTH

We briefly touched on the benefits collagen can offer toward your muscles, but let's go more in depth now. One of the main ways that collagen contributes to muscle growth is by enabling the body to produce creatine more efficiently (Muscleblaze, 2019). Creatine is made up of the amino acids within collagen, and is needed for muscle growth. As you work to gain muscles during exercise, your muscles need energy to grow, which is called ATP. ATP cannot develop without creatine, meaning that if your body has a decreased or insufficient level of creatine, your muscle growth will be far less noticeable. Making sure that your body has a higher level of creatine will give the body more energy to expend towards growing those muscles you are working so hard for.

Beyond that, collagen is also able to target the muscles and provide them with benefits in a more direct way. Studies have shown that collagen is effective at both relaxing and growing the blood vessels, which means much more needed oxygen is able to reach your muscles. This aids in the muscle recovery and building processes too. Collagen can also soothe muscle pain and damage, as well as provide the body with more tissues that muscle growth requires. Therefore, incorporating a collagen supplement into your workout diet is a great way to make sure that your body is generating enough of all of the resources it needs to allow you to bulk up your body with ease.

In this chapter, we covered the vast amount of benefits collagen can have on the body. There are so many benefits collagen provides that it is a wonder that everyone does not take it already. Collagen heals and protects the body in so many ways; it is a supplement to revere and including it in your diet is, in my opinion, one of the best things that you can do to boost your personal health. Next up, we are going to talk about exactly how to include collagen in your diet–you will learn about all the different forms of the supplement available as well as the best ways to take collagen so that you can decide what is right for you.

3

HOW TO TAKE COLLAGEN SUPPLEMENTS

C ollagen comes in a variety of forms, so it can be hard to determine which is the best for you if you are not aware of all of the potential options. Each supplement and each type is bound to have different advantages and disadvantages, and deciding on which one can or will work best for you with no prior knowledge is quite a challenge. As with any supplement, knowing when, how, and with what to take it is at all times an important consideration before beginning a dietary supplement. Your goal with any supplement is to make it part of your routine, and you are unable to do that without the valuable background information needed! In this chapter, we will cover all of this and more in depth. First, we are going to talk about the different forms of collagen.

FORMS OF COLLAGEN

In short, the most common ways to take a collagen supplement include pills, powders, bars, shots, liquid drinks, and gummies. Each type of the supplement is available over the counter or online, and they range from incredibly cheap to very expensive depending on your standards. There is something available for every age, gender, and budget to try when it comes to collagen supplements. Finding what works for you is all a matter of product research and a little dedication.

Collagen pills come like most other vitamin supplements do. That is, you can buy them over the counter in the nutritional section of any grocery store. A lot of collagen supplements have a blend of collagen and vitamin C, which is a great option for your health. Collagen gummies are an option as well, just like multivitamin gummies are. If you are looking for a quick way to ingest your collagen, a pill or gummy form might be best for you. These forms can be taken whenever you take your other supplements, medication, or eat your breakfast, making them a perfect addition to a routine. With these supplements, you will want to be sure to read the ingredients. Later on I will provide some helpful tips for making sure that your collagen supplement is not only pure, but free from anything unnatural or harmful as well, so it's good to know now that you are going to need to read those labels and read them well!

Collagen can also be purchased in shots or drinks, as well as be added to drinks yourself. Shots of collagen can be purchased relatively cheap online and work wonders to boost energy on account of all the vitamins they contain. You can also buy drinks with collagen or mix collagen powder into a drink yourself. This is a good option for people who struggle with taking pill forms of supplements but also lack the time to make a full meal or beverage with a blended collagen powder. You can simply open the shot up and drink it before going on with your day. Just like with the pills, though, we are going to need to check for ingredients.

Collagen powder is another way to take collagen, and it is probably the most popular method of taking collagen. Plus, this is the method I most endorse because of the fact that I have had the best experience with it; collagen powders can be far easier to absorb, contain higher levels of collagen per serving, and are a great way to incorporate your supplement into your daily routine. It is best to mix collagen into water by stirring it, but you can also include your collagen powder in coffee or tea. Implementing collagen powder as a part of your routine is best provided that you make it a part of something you already do. You can mix collagen powder with nearly anything you want, including all sorts of drinks like juice and smoothies, kombucha, hot chocolate, or anything else. You can also mix collagen powder into soft foods like yogurt. It is really not hard to add a collagen powder to your diet because it is such a versatile option.

For those who prefer a more food-based method of taking their collagen, most grocery stores also sell collagen bars. They come in packages just like protein bars and can make an awesome snack for work or school, supplement, work out snack, or part of a meal. You will want to check the ingredients labels thoroughly and purchase them in packs for the best price. This can be an incredibly convenient option for those of you who travel frequently, snack often, find yourself hungry often, or otherwise just want to swap out some junk food for a more healthy option. Finding a good tasting and collagen-rich snack bar to include in your pantry or lunchbox is sure to make a positive change in your life.

There are also some general things to keep in mind regarding your collagen supplement and which form you would prefer. If you want something pure and simple, I would suggest a collagen powder or pill. Shots, gummies, and bars are the best way to take collagen especially if you struggle with taking pills, especially if you're strapped for time, but be careful to make sure that these supplements actually contain a solid amount of collagen for the price. It is also important to be incredibly watchful if you are vegan, vegetarian, or follow other dietary restrictions. Many collagen supplements contain animal derivatives or hidden gelatin ingredients, which can be problematic for many diets. If you do follow a more restrictive diet, it might be easier to find a pill or powder form of a supplement to suit your needs.

BEST WAYS TO TAKE COLLAGEN

Collagen supplements can be taken at any time of day, although most professionals recommend taking it in the morning if you expect to experience energy-related benefits. Energy-related benefits are possible, but not common, and if you think you might get a bit of an energy kick from your supplement, it is good to start in the morning. Taking collagen at night has been linked to improved sleep and some people do find themselves tired after starting new supplements, so it is really up to you whether you take the collagen supplements you choose as a part of your morning routine or your nighttime routine. Ideally, you should aim for 5-10 grams of collagen a day for the best benefits. You can take as low as 2.5 grams and as much as 15 depending on various factors we will talk about in a bit, but for most people that 5-10 gram range is the sweet spot. It may seem better or tempting to you to take more, but I recommend avoiding this behavior–an excess of collagen can leave you with a myriad of health problems and negative side effects that I assure that you do not want to suffer.

A lot of people who are just starting out in their journey with collagen worry about heating up their collagen to consume it. Many foods are known to lose some of their nutritional value when you heat them up, especially if you use the microwave to do so, but collagen is not like that. Collagen maintains all of its nutrition even if you mix it into coffee or tea because it has a large amount of concentrated amino acids. Unless you plan to heat your collagen to a temperature that rivals that of lava, you are all good to heat it up. The temperature of boiling water is far below the maximum temperature for collagen, so I promise your collagen is safe in a tea or coffee.

Something else collagen newbies might think about is split dosing their supplement. If you are new to taking collagen supplements, you might find it best to split your dose up throughout the day. Scientifically, splitting the dose does not necessarily increase effectiveness in any way, nor does it lower it, but collagen is a protein nonetheless, and if you are not used to having sufficient protein in your body it can cause bloating initially. Some people also experience mild levels of drowsiness due to the sudden influx of nutrients that the body is not used to, but this is also a rare side effect. Overall, splitting the dose up at first is a good way to get your body used to collagen supplements, especially if you're sensitive to supplements or worried about side effects.

Personally, I would recommend collagen powder over any other form of the supplement to anyone who asks. Collagen powder is more easily absorbed than collagen in other forms, allowing you to reap the benefits of your supplement more successfully. Later, I will touch on all of the different things you can mix collagen powder into (because that is worth dedicating its own section to alone), but let's move forward and talk about how to actually mix collagen powder. Yes, there is a right and a wrong way to do this! In the event that you do not mix your collagen powder well or thoroughly, nothing bad will necessarily occur, but you are making your collagen less effective because clumped up collagen is too thick to be absorbed easily by the body.

To get the most out of your collagen powder, an ideal option is a shaker bottle. This type of blending method helps break up clumps in the collagen powder and makes mixing much easier, regardless of whether you are on the go or just want to save some money after purchasing what might have been a quite expensive collagen supplement. Additionally, using a shaker bottle means that you will not have to spend as much money on a more expensive blender option since they can be purchased relatively cheaply; shaker bottles are available at any retail store for just a few dollars. Whether you are looking for an affordable way to improve your collagen intake or simply want something easy and convenient, purchasing a shaker bottle is definitely worth considering.

Blenders are the fastest and most effective way to blend a supplement like collagen powder into a food or drink if you have access to one, but blenders are obviously not the most portable and can be rather loud. For this reason, a shaker bottle or the next option might be better for you if you live in a shared space or have minimal countertop space to use. Regardless, blenders are a good option for if you use collagen powder as a part of a morning routine involving smoothies or blended foods.

A third option for mixing collagen powder is a frother, which works best for blending collagen powder into hot drinks. Many people own frothers now as is due to the fun they can add to a morning beverage. Frothers

COLLAGEN IS LIFE | 61

can be used for far more than just your collagen
powder if you're creative enough. If you do not have
any of these options, a spoon will do the trick just fine.
Worst case, in the case that you do go with a spoon to
stir, you may experience significant amounts of clumping, or you might be stirring for a while. I definitely
recommend investing in a better blending tool in the
event that you choose to go with collagen powder over
pills.

Another important way to make sure that you are
taking your collagen in the best way possible is to make
sure that you have picked the right product for you,
your needs, and your routine. You cannot simply go
grab things off the shelf and expect magic to occur; you
have to know what you are doing before you hit those
shelves. In a later chapter I will describe in detail how
to choose the right supplement, and it really is a key
part of ensuring that your collagen routine is effective. I
truly cannot overstate how important the right supplement is. Besides, if you begin purchasing products at
random without knowing what you need, you are guaranteed to waste money that you could have otherwise
better placed elsewhere. You do not have any opportu-
nity to go wrong with starting off by knowing what
you need.

Furthermore, it is important to make sure that your collagen is actually blended well. I have put so much emphasis on blending collagen powder for good reason. That is, poorly blended collagen will not be absorbed as easily. The benefit of a collagen powder is that the powder can be completely dissolved into a food or liquid, so leaving clumps in your mixture is going to negate that benefit entirely. My recommendation is that if you are making a cold drink, blend the collagen up into a small amount of lukewarm or hot water before incorporating that into the final beverage. Some collagen powders do blend well in cold temperatures, but the best practice for mixing up collagen is to use at least room temperature water to do so. Otherwise, make sure your collagen powder is completely clump-free and you are good to go!

I also recommend putting yourself on a subscription service for your collagen supplement as well. Most companies you can order collagen from on the internet offer a subscription service, and Amazon even has their own "subscribe and save" option. These services charge your card monthly or every few months and send you the product automatically. I suggest opting into this because once you start a supplement, it can be incredibly easy to stop simply due to being too lazy to reorder the product. Under the circumstance that it comes to your door automatically, you will be more likely to continue your collagen routine for years to come. Also, it's usually more cost effective to subscribe to products instead of buying them individually every time you need them, so subscribing to a product you love is a win-win here.

The last thing to know pertaining to the most effective way to take collagen is how to allow your supplement to work best. In other words, it is important to know what you need to do outside of collagen supplementation to allow your body to best absorb and use those supplements effectively. Drinking tons of water and cutting down on sugar are the two best ways to increase the effectiveness of your supplement. If you do not drink water with your collagen, you may face dehydration, and sugar can damage the collagen in your body so it is best to avoid added sugars in your food and drinks. Collagen is a superhero of a supplement, and small amounts of sugar thus will not hurt your progress, but I definitely encourage making positive dietary changes to nudge your collagen supplement in the right direction as you begin this process.

With this information, you are all set to begin picking out collagen supplements. Keeping in mind form, type, and best practices for taking your supplement is key in making sure that you buy a product that will allow you to experience all of the benefits that we discussed previously. Also, I have not forgotten about natural alternatives to boosting your collagen levels either. It is definitely possible that you prefer natural boosts to your collagen instead of supplements, so that is what the next chapter will focus on–natural ways to aid the collagen production of your body and that do not rely on supplements.

4

HOW TO OBTAIN COLLAGEN NATURALLY

Taking collagen supplements can seem a bit redundant in our society; at all times, everyone is recommending something new for you to take in the name of health, so how can you even start to discern what your body actually needs? Contrary to a lot of what is being advertised online, collagen is one of the supplements and nutrients that your body absolutely cannot do without. Collagen improvement is not even solely based on supplements–collagen is one of the most abundant, natural things in our body, and as such, you can work to boost your collagen solely through making improvements to your diet. This means that supplements are completely unnecessary in case you want to go a more natural route with your collagen journey. Ideally, you will want to combine an approach of supplementation and lifestyle changes if you're hoping to experience the most fulfilling and extensive benefits collagen has to offer.

WHAT IS A COLLAGEN DIET?

A collagen diet is a great way to naturally boost the levels of collagen in your body without relying on supplements. It might sound as if a collagen diet encourages you to eat a significant amount of collagen, but that is not what a collagen diet intends for you to do at all. Instead, a collagen diet relies on certain food products–natural ones you probably already eat at least sometimes–to kick your collagen production levels up a notch. This is a more natural way to improve your collagen levels that can allow the body to absorb nutrients to a higher degree of efficiency than with supplements.

A collagen diet is one that emphasizes eating in a way that both prevents the degradation of collagen as well as allows for more collagen to be generated in the body (Davis, 2022). Namely, a collagen diet does this by avoiding sugary foods that can cause the breakdown of natural collagen stores, as well as by avoiding refined carbohydrates. Sugars and refined carbs both are good to avoid if you are serious about experiencing the benefits of a collagen diet. They lower or reduce the ability of your body to create, protect, and store collagen by causing a sudden spike in the insulin levels within the body, which then results in inflammation, and as you know by now, inflammation is no good for your collagen.

Collagen diets also encourage you to consume foods that are high in collagen themselves. As a part of a collagen diet, many people do opt to incorporate a mix of collagen-rich foods alongside collagen supplements in their preferred form, but this is not a requirement to working towards building a collagen-friendly diet. From my personal experience, I absolutely recommend working on developing healthy lifestyle habits which combine exercise, nutrition, and supplements to achieve your collagen-related goals.

Collagen-friendly foods that are usually added to a collagen diet span a variety of food groups and items. The foods recommended for participants in collagen dieting all aim to target improved skin elasticity and joint pain, and are said to possess anti-aging properties as well. Meats that contain high levels of collagen include fish and chicken, and as far as proteins go, egg whites are a viable option for collagen as well. You should make sure to avoid processed meat and all processed food in general for your health; fresh fish and chicken are going to provide you with those desirable collagen boosts. Processed food has little to no nutritional value whatsoever. Vegetables like leafy greens, peppers, and beans are good additions to the diet, as well as fruits like avocado and tomato. Berries, citrus, and white tea are also high in collagen. You can also consider nuts like cashews too. Many keto diets are prone to provide people with healthy collagen stores because of the foods they promote and the foods they encourage you to avoid.

It is important to note that if you are vegan, you might have to approach collagen dieting and supplementation in a way that is more streamlined to your diet. Chicken and fish are obviously not vegan, and since supplements are often made from the bodies of animals, it can be a bit discouraging to look for collagen supplements as a vegan. I am glad I get to break this news to you–it is possible to lead a collagen-friendly, vegan diet! Science has found a way to develop vegan collagen supplements that avoid using animal products, including gelatin, altogether (Reisdorf, 2019). Combined with a strong dietary base, vegans and other people on stricter diets can safely and confidently access the benefits a collagen diet has to offer.

So, how is it possible for a vegan collagen supplement to be produced? The process through which this ability was discovered was initially rather complicated, but the process can be broken down in simple to understand terms. While studying the bacteria that collagen requires to successfully function, researchers have discovered that a bacteria called *P. pastoris* is the most effective bacteria that is used to synthetically engineer the best quality collagen. In order to use these bacteria, human gene codes that correlate to collagen were added to the bacteria in a lab, which then turns into human collagen. After that, the digestive enzyme pepsin is added to the mix in order to allow the synthetic collagen to resemble human collagen more closely. This entirely genetically modified collagen is made 100% free of animal products, making it a perfectly vegan option for collagen supplementation. Remember, not all genetic modification is bad, but you should look carefully into how and with what your collagen is genetically modified if you are opting to trust a genetically modified or GMO product.

You might be wondering now how vegan collagen measures up to non-vegan collagen. Vegan collagen actually has a plethora of benefits in its own right. For starters, lab produced collagen may be a cheaper alternative to collagen that is originally sourced from animals or uses animal components as a primary ingredient. Vegan collagen also lowers the risk of allergen contamination or general allergic reactions to collagen; one of the most important considerations when buying a collagen supplement is, after all, whether you are allergic to the ingredients. Opting for a vegan-friendly collagen supplement if you are prone to allergies relating to typical collagen ingredients may allow the process of selecting a supplement to go much smoother. Lab developed collagen also has the potential to be safer due to the highly controlled environment in which it is produced. Vegan, lab developed collagen offers all of the same benefits as animal sourced collagen while providing a handful of unique benefits that give consumers ample control in their supplement choices. There is really no reason to worry that a vegan collagen alternative is less beneficial than a non-vegan one, so if you are a vegan looking for a collagen supplement, or if you are incredibly sensitive to many supplements available on the market, there are absolutely safe options for you as well.

Regarding natural, food-based options for vegans, many of the options listed above for non-vegans will work as well. In place of products like chicken or fish, you can incorporate more soy products into your diet, as well as legumes and practically any nut or seed you can like. Any food or recipe that calls for chicken or fish can easily be swapped out for tofu and prepared in the same manner, because tofu is a phenomenal source of protein that helps support the development of collagen. Tofu is a great option for anyone on a diet that can result in lower levels of protein in the body, and it makes a tasty addition to any dish if you know what you are doing. You can also benefit from amino acid supplements since these are more abundant and easy to find in stores than vegan collagen supplements are as of yet. Amino acid supplements are also a good way to boost collagen levels by taking the amino acids that the body uses to build collagen itself. Furthermore, ensuring that you consume a diet rich in tomatoes, berries, and dark, leafy greens will put you on a level playing field with any meat eater collagen wise; you just have to become an expert on what your options are.

WAYS TO BOOST NATURAL GROWTH OF COLLAGEN

Outside of food-based options, there are plenty of other ways to supplement the growth of your body's collagen naturally. This includes both other supplements as well as simple lifestyle changes that your body will appreciate and be able to produce and protect your collagen as an end result of. In other words, adding non-collagen supplements to your daily routine can provide your collagen levels with some added support, and you can also incorporate other products and habits into your life that are great for collagen.

For example, adding hyaluronic acid supplements is not only fantastic for your skin, but also helps the collagen in your body as well. Hyaluronic acid allows water to bind to collagen, which provides aid to the hydrating qualities that collagen offers. This, in turn, allows your skin to maintain elasticity. Hydration is vital to your collagen levels as I have mentioned before, and if your skin is not sensitive adding hyaluronic acid to your skincare routine is a good idea as well. However, be sure that you are not going to have a severe reaction to any new skin products you try because that is very counterintuitive. If you are not wanting to take a collagen supplement directly, ensuring that your body has enough hyaluronic acid is one of the next best things.

Vitamin C is another helpful supplement to take in lieu of collagen supplements. There is a reason many collagen supplements also contain vitamin C; vitamin C keeps your collagen strong and functioning by preventing the enzymes in collagen from becoming inactive. Overall, vitamin C is good for helping your body produce more collagen than it does, and it protects the existing collagen in your body from degradation. This mostly impacts collagen type I. Vitamin C supplements or the inclusion of more vitamin C containing foods–such as oranges–is a great way to boost collagen production in the body. The value of

vitamin C to collagen stores cannot be overstated–
these benefits are why so many supplements combine
collagen and vitamin C into one pill. If you do not
already have a vitamin C supplement or make sure that
you consume enough vitamin C on a daily basis,
starting to do so now is instrumental in allowing your
collagen diet or supplement to have its full effect.

Something else you can utilize to stimulate your
collagen is, surprisingly, aloe vera gel. Lotion,
sunscreen, or other skin products containing aloe vera
gel are fantastic for collagen, because it stimulates the
ability of your body to produce collagen. Plenty of
drinks are available containing aloe vera gel as well,
and they come in so many flavors that you are guaranteed to find one you love. Much like hyaluronic acid,
aloe vera gel improves the elasticity of your skin, which
explains why it is a key ingredient in many skin products. Aloe is also good at binding skin cells in a way that
softens and smooths them. Aloe vera gel and products
containing aloe are a good addition to your skincare
regimen to consider if you are hoping to boost collagen
without taking a collagen supplement directly.

Ginseng and antioxidants are two more nutritional
components for the diet of anyone wanting a natural
supplement to their collagen. Ginseng is incredibly
natural and contains many vitamins, including D and

B12. Ginseng is also able to create better circulation throughout the body, thus boosting oxygen levels and collagen along with it. You can find ginseng at the store in teas or in its most natural form; a root. This can be added to dishes, your own teas, etc., to provide benefits to your collagen stores. Antioxidants work amazingly for supporting collagen too. Antioxidants come in many forms and work to protect your collagen tissues by reducing the amount of free radicals in your body. Free radicals–unstable atoms that can damage cells and tissues–are known to speed up the process of collagen degradation. Antioxidants can also speed up the process of producing new collagen.

Furthermore, retinol is a good way to promote the development of collagen. It works similarly to other solutions mentioned; collagen stores grow because of retinol's ability to stimulate the necessary cells responsible for its growth. Retinol is in a vast amount of skin-care products as well as oral supplements, often the main selling point for them, as retinol has the ability to provide elasticity for your skin and works to slow or reverse the aging process. Red light therapy works similarly. For the duration of red-light therapy, your skin is exposed to high levels of red light that are said to be absorbed by the mitochondria. The mitochondria then uses the light absorbed from this form of therapy

COLLAGEN IS LIFE | 75

to produce more energy, which, in turn, leads to increased collagen production.

One more important natural aspect of protecting and increasing your bodily collagen is to protect your skin from nature. Specifically, it is best to make sure that your skincare routine includes a sunscreen with an SPF of at least 30 in order to prevent UV rays emitted by the sun from damaging your skin. Overlooking sunscreen and protecting your skin from the environment is one major way people contribute to the deterioration of their health without even noticing. You can also protect your skin from the environment by taking care of the level of moisture your skin retains if you expose it to dry climates often.

All of these solutions are ways that you can benefit the amount of collagen in your body, especially as you age. Scientifically, these solutions work by stimulating something called "fibroblasts." These are a form of cell responsible for growing the connective tissues that make up your joints, tendons, and more. Fibroblasts release collagen as a byproduct, and things like retinol, aloe, and vitamin C do wonders for making sure that your fibroblasts work properly. Implementing one or multiple of the above techniques is sure to allow your collagen to work to keep your body healthy and skin vibrant.

FOODS THAT HELP YOUR BODY PRODUCE COLLAGEN

We have talked about supplement and dietary options for boosting collagen without taking collagen, so now it is time to go over the best way to supplement your collagen levels with some good, plain food. For many people, it might be a bit confusing that anyone would opt for a food-based solution to their collagen levels since there are pills that seem to take care of the whole process. It is actually rather common, and even good, for you to approach health concerns with food first and foremost.

For starters, the body is typically able to process fresh fruits and vegetables as well as unprocessed, lean meats more easily than a manufactured supplement. For generations, we survived without supplements because we had to make do with food, so it's what the body is more ready to absorb and utilize. Then, relying on natural foods is a good way to weed out potential allergies and sensitivities that you could experience with collagen supplements if you are not careful. You have been eating food for your entire life, so you likely know by now what you are and are not allergic to, or at least what makes you feel unwell when you eat it. That said, chances are you are a lot less familiar with what supplements are okay for you to digest, so starting with natural food options might be better for you. Not everything needs an actual supplement, pill, gummy, or special drink–collagen can be helped by increasing the levels of certain foods you eat, most of which you probably already have in your fridge or buy regularly anyway.

There are plenty of options for food options you can choose from to provide your body with a collagen boost. As I have briefly mentioned earlier, some of the best foods you can include in your diet for supporting your natural collagen include chicken, fish, and egg whites (Marengo, 2019). Many collagen supplements are sourced from chicken and other lean meats and proteins, so what better way to supplement collagen with food than by starting with chicken. Chicken contains a massive amount of collagen, and studies have shown that the cartilage found in chicken has been effective for relieving arthritic pains. Collagen is also found in the meat of fish, and while egg whites are not collagen-rich, they can help your body develop collagen too. You can consume the yolk of the egg too, but that is not bound to provide you with any collagen-related benefits. Swapping out your red meat products for chicken is an awesome way to use food to your advantage when it comes to collagen.

Fish and certain other marine life are a good source of natural, food-based collagen as well because the bones, ligaments, and overall, most of the body of seafood creatures is composed of collagen. It is important to note, however, that the main fish meat you are used to is not the most collagen-rich part of the fish. Because of this, it is best to use fish as a supplement in combination with other food items, as eating copious amounts of fish is not actually good for you. Just eating more fish alone probably will not do you much good with regard to your collagen levels or maintenance. Still, swapping out your red meat for a combination of fish and chicken is an excellent way to make a food based change to your collagen levels.

Egg whites are also in this family of collagen-rich foods because of their status as an animal product. Contrary to most animal products, though, egg whites themselves do not contain collagen because they contain no connective tissues. Instead, egg whites are rich in protein which builds up collagen in a unique way compared to many other animal products. For this reason, swapping egg whites with soy and other plant based forms of protein is a valid way for vegetarians, vegans, or anyone else who is avoiding certain animal products to reap the benefits of food-based collagen supplementation. A good amount of protein in your diet goes a long way in improving your health.

COLLAGEN IS LIFE | 79

Something else you can do to aid in the ability of your body to produce collagen is to consume lots of vitamin C. This means citrus fruits should play a significant role in your everyday dietary choices. Fruits, like oranges and grapefruits, are an awesome choice for breakfast, and lemons and limes can be good for vitamin C too. If you are on certain medications, be careful of consuming grapefruit though; grapefruit can cause unwanted reactions with medications. Did you know tomatoes are filled with vitamin C as well? We consume tomatoes in so many foods on a daily basis, but most people do not know that tomatoes contain nearly 30% of the vitamin C that your body needs to create collagen. Also, berries are also a phenomenal source of vitamin C. Contrary to popular belief, strawberries tend to be more rich in vitamin C than oranges are. Other berries are great for boosting your levels of vitamin C as well. Beyond that, due to the antioxidant properties of many berries, they also serve the dual purpose of protecting your collagen from degradation due to the free radicals I mentioned earlier. Berries can be added to yogurt or other breakfast foods or just eaten as a snack–they are a simple and tasty dietary inclusion to help your body out with collagen production and maintenance.

As it turns out, garlic is a great way to boost your body's collagen production too. Garlic is a beloved ingredient in many dishes, and it packs more of a punch than just flavor. Due to the high sulfur content found within garlic, garlic is able to help produce and prevent the breakdown of collagen. We have been talking about a lot of aspects surrounding the building up of more collagen, but it is just as important to keep the collagen you do have from deteriorating due to various circumstances. Unfortunately, you do need a lot of garlic to see benefits to your collagen levels, so it is best to combine garlic with other foods known to boost collagen. Still, garlic is a great addition to anyone's diet because it has so many benefits beyond just flavor and collagen. If you are a fan of garlic, do not be afraid to add extra to any recipe that calls for it!

Vegetarians and vegans reading many of the items on this list may be concerned, once again, that it is difficult or impossible to reap the benefits of a food-based, collagen-friendly diet. That said, there is no reason to worry because there are many more available food options that are a good fit for your dietary needs. For example, leafy greens like spinach and kale are amazing for supporting collagen. Chlorophyll is something that is a key player in the makeup of any green plant–it is what gives the plant its color! Chlorophyll is naturally an antioxidant, giving it the same benefit towards protecting collagen from free radicals as many berries. A combined approach of plentiful berries, vitamin C, and chlorophyll is going to inundate your body with the resources it needs to do great things with your collagen levels. Ensuring that your diet contains sufficient amounts of dark, leafy greens is a perfect way for anyone, regardless of dietary restriction, to benefit from the collagen-related support that food has to offer.

As far as further food options go, beans and legumes are also among the list of vegan- and vegetarian-friendly collagen boosting food options. Beans not only contain the amino acids that your body needs to produce collagen, but they are also rich in copper. Without copper, your body cannot produce sufficient collagen either, meaning you should try to include beans into your diet too. If you are not a fan of beans, you can try cashews instead, or vice versa. Cashews have both zinc and copper in them, making them a stellar choice for boosting collagen production in the body. It is important to ensure that your body gets all of these essential vitamins and minerals in order to elevate your collagen levels naturally.

And finally, do not be afraid to leverage a multivitamin or specific individual vitamin supplements to your advantage. It is not uncommon that someone's diet will lack something like zinc, vitamin C, copper, etc., or a combination of several of these minerals. Be it due to allergy, inaccessible resources for those minerals, or anything else causing you to potentially have lower than ideal levels of vitamins and minerals necessary to collagen production, a multivitamin or individual vitamin can save the day. If you find yourself lacking nutritional options from food, finding supplementary options can help meet your nutrition halfway on providing your body what it needs.

MEAL IDEAS FOR COLLAGEN SUPPORT

Knowing what foods to use to boost your collagen levels is undoubtedly a great help, but what good is a list of food without some ideas for meals, right? I am not by any means here to provide you with a comprehensive cookbook, but I do have some recommendations for meals that you can try out to include collagenated foods into your diet. Some phenomenal meals you can create with collagen-boosting foods include:

- Skin-on chicken with carrots and broccoli. Eating chicken with the skin on is at all times a far preferable option because that means you are consuming the collagen from the skin of the chicken directly. Chicken skin is an immaculate source of collagen, and the vegetables paired with the chicken in this dish do wonders to further boost collagen production. This is a common dish recommended for a variety of benefits, so you can definitely find a recipe you like online.

- Spinach salad. Incorporating chicken, berries, eggs, or other collagen boosting foods into your salad is a great food option for those looking to make collagen-rich meals.
- Sardine or chicken pasta. Fettuccine or other pasta based meals with sardines or chicken in them are a good way to boost your collagen production. Adding in a garnish of diced tomatoes or red peppers will give the dish some extra vitamins as well.
- Smoothies full of berries, which you can also mix your collagen powder into.
- Chia pudding with berries.
- Beef or chicken bone broth. Cows and chicken are both good sources of collagen for humans, and bone broths provide benefits without any potential drawbacks of red meats. Using bone broth for soups or other meals will give you a nice additional source of collagen in your meals.
- Any food with gelatin in it. For the most part, these consist of candies, so opting for natural or

sugar-free candies is a good idea, but gelatin is, in and of itself, a very abundant source of collagen.

Those are just a few ideas of what you can make to start incorporating collagen-friendly foods into your regular meal planning. If you crave something else or want to try out more meal ideas, looking up "collagen-boosting meal ideas" with your preferred search engine will grant you hundreds of options. You can mix and match ideas and foods and find out which recipes are your favorite, and soon you'll be eating a collagen diet without even having to think about it.

HERBAL REMEDIES

For a lot of people, herbal remedies feel like a more soothing and natural way to approach supplementing their body with the nutrients that they need, and collagen is no different. Natural supplements are another powerful option and luckily, herbal remedies are plentiful regarding what you can do to benefit the collagen supply of your body and collagen development. Personally, I do not have much experience with all of the herbal remedies that contribute to bettering collagen in the body, as this is not something I am heavily interested in; however, I have researched colla-

COLLAGEN IS LIFE | 85

gen-friendly herbal remedies extensively to have the background knowledge and have a few great herbal remedies in mind that you can try if a more herbal approach is more suited to you and your tastes.

Before taking any herbal supplement, be sure to do appropriate research into the side effects, medical warnings, and drug interactions involved. I cannot express enough the importance of verifying whether or not an herbal option is safe for you before you include it in your diet. Many herbs can interact negatively with medications, have bad effects toward pregnancy, and can otherwise make you feel drowsy or unwell, and it is non-negotiable to research herbs you plan to put into your body carefully if you want to ensure your own safety.

With that being said, horsetail is one herb that is good for your collagen levels (Team, 2019). In its stem, horsetail is rife with magnesium, potassium, and calcium, as well as silica. Silica, while not directly helpful to collagen, can improve connective tissues which helps collagen do the job it is supposed to. Horsetail is also an herb that is incredibly easily absorbed by the body, making it a great choice. You can turn horsetail into a tea or take it in capsule form. You can also eat horsetail raw, but it has no taste this way. Nettles are also good for collagen because they serve as a multivitamin with a high concentration of many essential vitamins that the body needs to produce collagen. On their own, nettles can improve the hair, bones, immune system, and many of the body's organs, and the nutrients in nettles are sure to provide your body with anything you are missing from being able to develop collagen. Another herb you can try is calendula, which is easier to find for most people than the other two. Topical application of calendula is scientifically and medically supported, which means that it can provide similar effects to collagen or assist topical collagen treatment in healing wounds at an escalated rate.

Those are just a few of the many examples of herbs that you can try for elevating collagen levels. A brief list of others you can try includes:

- turmeric
- gingko
- basil
- rosemary
- aloe
- oregano
- amla
- comfrey
- marigold
- burdock

For the above herbs, you have several options for what you can do with them in order to aid the collagen levels in your body. The most common way people utilize herbs like the ones above is in tea. Purchasing an organic bag of the herb, for example, and steeping it in a tea ball is a good way to make a natural tea from an herb directly. You can also buy teas that come with those herbs, some of which are far easier to find than others, or blend several of your herbs together and make your own tea. Another option is finding a capsule for the herb, which is not that hard at all due to the rising popularity of herbal supplementation. I also recommend aloe vera drinks and topical creams, along with topical creams involving other herbs on that list if you think that is something you would personally benefit from trying.

There is not a lot of extensive evidence supporting the idea that herbs are directly beneficial to collagen, but there is plenty that supports other uses of herbal remedies. Using herbs to increase vitamins, minerals, and other compounds in the body, as well as creating certain desired effects in the body such as relaxation, can indirectly benefit the protection and development of your collagen. It is a well-known fact that various teas, creams, and other herbal practices can benefit the body in a myriad of ways, and I do not see why this can't extend into collagen supplementation. So, even if you are not getting collagen directly from the herb, you can still supplement your collagen growth in other ways. If you prefer herbal options for collagen supplement, the bottom line is that there are plentiful options for you as well.

DESTRESSING FOR YOUR COLLAGEN'S SAKE

I mentioned earlier in the book how elevated stress levels impact collagen levels–stress causes inflammation which also raises cortisol, and then our body is unable to produce the collagen it needs. With a world so inundated with stress and obligation, it can be hard to find a way to relax, but if you find yourself constantly overwhelmed and stressed or feel yourself approaching a breaking point, it may be time to focus on relaxation. Stress does play a role in speeding up the aging process, so I would encourage you to find ways to rest and relax.

In order to focus on relaxation, you first need to find a technique that works for you. You can opt for anything so long as it does not create more stress in your life. Meditation is one way that you can work on relaxing the body. Meditation works by allowing the breathing to slow down and the mind to dissolve all worries, at least temporarily. If done correctly, you will also experience plentiful muscle relaxation that can, on its own, do wonders to alleviate pain. If you are interested in meditating to alleviate stress, YouTube guided meditations can be a lifesaver. Otherwise, just focus on clearing your mind and paying attention to your breathing, and you will feel far calmer after a few minutes. Counting to 10 slowly, the old trick parents use to soothe themselves, does actually work!

Something else I would recommend is yoga or other light exercise in addition to your usual exercise regimen. Instead of focusing on the rate at which your heart is beating, finding a soothing exercise like yoga or walking can be a good way to lower cortisol and stress. Paying attention to your body and where it is and what it is doing is a very soothing process. In the next section, I will talk about exercises that boost your level of collagen production, but that is not what I mean to do for relaxation. Instead, for relaxation, you are going to want to focus on any exercise that encourages deep breathing, stretching, and a sense of calm.

Another way you can work toward relaxation in order to help your body return to producing the collagen it should is to find a creative outlet you enjoy. Journalling, art, music, or any other hobby, can be shockingly stress-relieving. Hobbies are known to be a great way to alleviate stress while simultaneously allowing for self-expression, and if you do not already have a go-to hobby, I do suggest finding one you enjoy partaking in on a regular basis.

You can also generally work to avoid factors in your life that cause inflammation because inflammation and stress go hand in hand. If you experience significant amounts of joint inflammation, for example, elevating the joints, and otherwise working to reduce the physical inflammation you experience, is a good way to encourage along collagen growth. Furthermore, if you are someone who experiences high levels of stress or inflammation, I recommend cutting out spicy foods, sugars, sodium, and bread where necessary, because all of these food options contribute to inflammation.

Again, destressing to reduce inflammation and related bodily issues is something that I and many other collagen experts consider to be vital to the process of developing a healthy level of collagen in the body, as well as protecting your current levels of collagen. Inflammation caused in the body due to stress is not your friend in any capacity, and you should really avoid inflammation at all costs. Finding ways to maintain a lower level of stress, cortisol, or inflammation will go a long way in providing you with countless collagen-related benefits.

EXERCISE FOR COLLAGEN PRODUCTION

Another natural form of increasing the level of collagen your body produces is to leverage exercise to your benefit. Many studies have shown that not only is exercise amazing for increasing collagen production levels, but it can also aid in the process of recovery or healing from various physical ailments. Not just any exercise is going to boost your collagen levels though; it is important to know the specifics.

Collagen increases due to exercise when the strength necessary for an exercise is greater than what the body is typically "able" to handle. In other words, if you are someone who has trained in improving muscles in the arms, you are going to need a far higher intensity of exercise to see collagen-related benefits as opposed to if you were working with your legs. This means that exercises like yoga, walking, or other light exercises, while good for your health, are extremely unlikely to have a marked or noticeable impact on improving the levels of collagen production in your body. Research suggests that the best form of exercise for collagen production is acute intensive exercise.

How did they come to this conclusion in the first place? Multiple studies have been conducted which showed marked increase in collagen production levels after the course of an acute intensive exercise training regimen; parts of the body that were not exercised did not appreciate any collagen-related benefits from the exercise. To read more about the impact of exercise alongside collagen treatment, skip ahead to the case studies section in Chapter 6, where I cover a variety of studies in depth, some of which cover exercise and training as well.

It is also important to know that, before beginning a collagen-boosting exercise routine, your exercise routine must be consistent. The studies involving the impact of exercise on collagen production levels are not nearly as extensive as in other areas pertaining to collagen, but the studies have concluded something vital: You have to keep exercising to see the benefits. Overwhelmingly, participants in these studies showed significant raises in collagen production levels for a few days after an exercise or consistent acute intensive workout routine, but those collagen levels declined once again after the exercise rituals stopped. Studies seem to be in accord that collagen production levels rise for three days after exercise and then stop rising at approximately five days. This is why it is important to commit to an exercise routine you will follow and take seriously. I do recommend exercise as a way to maintain overall health as well as to boost collagen, but it is absolutely essential that you make your exercise a habit.

Of course, before beginning your collagen boosting-exercise routine, you will need to know specifically what exercises to do as well as what acute intensive exercise is. For the most part, resistance and endurance training are included in acute exercise; do not worry if you are unfamiliar with these words. I am going to list a variety of exercises that fall under the category of 'acute intensive exercise' and that can be beneficial for aiding your body in collagen production. Another key component of acute intensive exercise is to get your heart rate up. A good goal range for your heart rate is 150-160 beats per minute, but this does vary per person. Getting your heart rate up during exercise is a known way to improve the quality of your workout—when you have an elevated heart rate, your blood and oxygen flow significantly better than when your heart beats at its normal, resting rate.

There are undoubtedly hundreds of potential exercises you can include in your exercise circuit or practice that meet these requirements. Though, I know it can be a bit daunting to begin a new exercise practice headfirst, so I want to make sure you have some specific examples and ideas to consider. Some heart rate-elevating resistance and/or endurance exercises that you can include into your workout routine are:

- Dumbbell exercises. There is a wide variety of dumbbell exercises that you can go for, all of which are good for resistance and strength training and may be beneficial to collagen levels. Some specific dumbbell maneuvers you might try include bicep curls, step ups, and the Arnold press.
- If you have access to a gym or workout machines in general, I recommend making use of them! Pull downs, leg presses, cable crossovers, and seated chest presses are just a few of the machine-based exercises that can be great for boosting your collagen levels.
- Reverse crunches. Reverse crunches are a great training method for collagen. In order to do a reverse crunch, you are going to need to lay down with your legs straight in front of you and your palms rested flat on the ground next to you. Ideally, your entire body will be flat at first so that you can experience the most benefit from this exercise. Cross your ankles over each other, and then, using your abdominal muscles, raise your legs up in the air. You should feel this exercise in your abdomen, and it will raise your hips up off the ground.
- Bicycle. No, not the thing with the pedals–this is the name of a fun and invigorating exercise as

well. To perform the bicycle, lay flat on the ground with your palms next to you. Bend your legs at a 90 degree angle, with your knees aligned above your hips. Make circular motions with your legs, as if you are pedaling a bicycle. For more of a challenge, you can elevate your hips with your hands and elbows, but be extremely careful when you do this.

These are just a few of the many examples of exercises you can incorporate into your routine to raise collagen levels. This is something I do suggest implementing as part of your new and improved, collagen-friendly life-style for your health generally as well as your collagen. Plus, strong muscles are never a bad thing.

It is absolutely possible to allow the collagen in your body to flourish in natural ways that do not rely on taking collagen supplements directly. Through a collagen-friendly diet, supplementing your collagen with other vitamins and such available over the counter, and keeping in mind foods and exercises that will help boost collagen levels while protecting your body's collagen, you can take a more natural approach to this journey. As you may already know though, too much of a good thing can turn into a bad thing. That is why this next chapter focuses on the potential negative side effects of taking collagen.

5

POTENTIAL SIDE EFFECTS OF TAKING COLLAGEN

W hen starting any new dietary change or routine, especially the inclusion of supplements into your diet, it is expected and even necessary to worry about potential side effects that the change can have. No one wants to start taking something they thought would be wonderful for them only to be suddenly struck with the realization that they have made themselves unwell in the process. That is why knowing the potential side effects and how to avoid them is essential when beginning the process of taking collagen.

Fortunately, collagen is a relatively safe thing to put in your body. It is such a significant player in keeping our bodies healthy and functional that it is near impossible to face negative side effects from taking collagen supplements. The only way that you are prone to suffer negative side effects from taking a collagen supplement is if you overdose on collagen. I mentioned earlier that 5-10 grams a day is the usual recommended dosage. However, that dose can vary depending on your age, activity level, and more. In just a brief moment, I am going to brief you on the majority of the common potential side effects of taking too much collagen. If you only take a 5-gram dose and experience those side effects as an end result, that may be a sign that you should wean yourself down to 2.5 grams. On the other hand, if you are a very active, 30-year-old athlete experiencing severe joint pain or injury, after starting with a 5-gram dose, you might find it beneficial to bump yourself to 15. It all depends on your lifestyle and body, and it is best to verify with your doctor that the way you are choosing to supplement your collagen levels is best for you.

It is very rare, therefore, that you will face any side effects from taking collagen. Overdosing on collagen is the only major risk outside of allergies that you can sustain from a collagen supplement, which is why it is so important to know what your correct dosage is and the potential side effects that you could encounter if you overdose on collagen. Beyond that, knowing the side effects can serve as a signal that you may need to lower your collagen dose or switch to a different prod-

COLLAGEN IS LIFE | 99

uct, so it's in your best interest to be aware of the side effects either way. To caution you sufficiently on what can happen if you do take too much collagen, I have provided below a myriad of the side effects that can stem from overdosing on collagen supplements.

One negative side effect you may face if you take collagen in excess is digestive issues like constipation or diarrhea. Overdosing on collagen can be incredibly dangerous, as it is known to cause gut health issues if taken in excess. This can cause the above issues as well as developing or worsening symptoms of IBS, so it is important to moderate your dosage well. Much like collagen can provide a reprieve from symptoms of IBS, it can also cause it. No one wants to suffer from gut health issues when taking a supplement intended to resolve them. If you are taking a collagen supplement and notice gut health or digestive health issues, that is a sure sign to either lower your collagen dose or to switch products. Persisting symptoms even after a product switch indicates that you are in fact taking too much collagen, in which case I would recommend halving your current dosage to see if symptoms subside.

As an end result of taking too much collagen, you may also be subject to poor appetite or bloating. The first few times you take collagen supplements, you can feel bloated or really full after taking it. This is because collagen is a protein and your body is breaking down amino acids in a level it is not used to. For most people, these symptoms dissipate once the body is used to the collagen supplement. In the case of people who over-dose on collagen supplements, however, this uneasy feeling of bloating can persist.

Kidney stones are another possible side effect that can occur as a result of taking collagen in amounts that exceed the recommended dosage. Kidney stones can be caused by collagen due to a high amount of the amino acid hydroxyproline. This amino acid is apt to be converted into a substance called oxalate, which is responsible for the development of kidney stones when it meets urine. Collagen-related kidney stones are not a common concern at all, because the levels of hydrox-yproline found within collagen are not typically high enough to cause kidney stones. However, if you take too much of your collagen supplement, you are at an increased risk of developing kidney stones as a result. People who are prone to developing kidney stones should also avoid collagen supplements or consult a doctor about the best way to progress in order to avoid these painful occurrences from forming.

High levels of calcium can also be a result of taking too much collagen. Many of us know calcium as the material responsible for making the bones stronger, but having too much calcium can actually cause your bones to deteriorate. High calcium can also be responsible for kidney stones and prevent your heart or brain from working as intended. It can be very hard to detect high levels of calcium in the body without medical intervention, and it might seem a bit odd to ask your doctor to check your calcium levels. As such, it is important to monitor your dosage and the presence of any other collagen-related and negative side effects; a myriad of other symptoms may indicate that you should reach out to your doctor for further advice on your collagen treatment options.

Another potential side effect of taking too much collagen is an allergic reaction. If you are allergic or sensitive to connective tissues, bones, or skin of animals, taking non-vegan collagen may not be for you. Some people have a natural sensitivity to collagen, which can cause the body to identify it as something that does not belong. The immune system then attacks the collagen supplement, making you incredibly ill as a result. It is essential to ensure that you have no underlying collagen sensitivities before taking a collagen supplement. Also, sometimes collagen supplements can result in breakouts or rashes. This is typically a result of collagen sensitivity and may indicate that you need to try a different source of collagen. If you do find that you are allergic to the collagen supplement you have selected, try a different brand or a supplement that offers different ingredients. Vegan collagen supplements are good for those with high levels of sensitivities, and opting for a lifestyle change works too, if you ultimately have a severe enough level of allergy that you cannot take any collagen supplement you find.

Liver fibrosis can also happen if you consume too much collagen. This can occur as a result of too much collagen type I in the liver and can decrease the ability of your liver to function properly. Liver fibrosis can be severe and even deadly, and it is not something that will be as immediately apparent as other symptoms. Once again, this just serves to exemplify why you should care to monitor the other symptoms of overdosing on collagen seriously.

Something you should at all times do as well is check the interactions between any new supplements you plan to take and any medication that you are currently on. Collagen supplements, or the ingredients they include, can sometimes interact negatively with different medications. Mood changes can result from overtaking collagen as well. My final piece of advice regarding the side effects that can result from collagen supplements is to consult a doctor if you have any questions or concerns. Collagen supplements are one

COLLAGEN IS LIFE | 103

of the safest things you can take, and your doctor will be able to help you out with any advice or adjustments as necessary. It's better to be safe than sorry medically, so make sure if you suspect anything to be wrong that you schedule a medical appointment as soon as possible.

As someone who has enjoyed the benefits of collagen supplements for years now, I can safely say that these side effects are nothing to worry about if you are careful and knowledgeable about how to take your collagen. It is possible that you might feel tempted to load up on collagen and account for lost time from just now learning about collagen and its abilities, but doing so is probably one of the worst ways you can begin your journey with taking collagen. Managing the amount you take above all and ensuring that you know what your body needs is the guaranteed way to avoid collagen-related side effects. As you can see, the side effects from collagen are few, but serious, and your health is nothing to play around with.

TAKING COLLAGEN SAFELY

There are lots of things to consider when learning how to safely begin your journey towards health with collagen. It is a simple enough process—you just need to make sure your dosage is right. Again, 2.5-15 grams per day is the sweet spot you should try to fall into, and you should start low even if you think you need a higher dose. Slowly increase your dose over the period of a few weeks if necessary.

You should also be sure to take the right type and do research into the brand you are taking. Make sure that the brand contains no allergens that can give you a bad reaction and find out what type of collagen the supplement you are looking at has. Look at all of the ingredients and research what they do as well. This is an especially important step for people who are vegan, kosher, or follow any other dietary guidelines–collagen sources can contain gelatin or other animal products that you need to avoid. Checking the ingredient labels and doing research for specific brands is vital before beginning any collagen supplement.

It is also a good idea to consult with a doctor if you are hesitant about a collagen supplement or have questions. Your doctor can help you decide which dosage is best for you, recommend products or lifestyle changes, and otherwise make the process run more smoothly. The two people who know your body best are you and your doctor, so combining your experience and their knowledge is the best way to go. Also, your doctor might even have some essential advice or recommendations for collagen-related habits that are better for your body than anything you can gain from a book, so I do suggest keeping your doctor in the loop about any major changes you make in your life towards your health, and that includes taking collagen.

I have told you all about the positive benefits, science, side effects, and other aspects of taking collagen, but the proof is in the pudding. Next, we are going to explore various case studies that have shown clear success in collagen related trials to show you how collagen is proven to be beneficial to the body in various ways, even under rigorous scientific study. If you still have hesitations about the benefits collagen can offer on a scientific level, I promise this next chapter will quell those concerns.

6

CASE STUDIES ON COLLAGEN

No supplement that shows as many benefits as collagen does can go unstudied. Hundreds, if not thousands, of collagen-related scientific experiments have been conducted over the years, many of which prove the benefits of collagen once and for all. If you are interested in evidence that collagen works, or if you are still hesitant about it working for you and your body, learning about some of the successful case studies involving collagen may help reassure you. Plus, learning about all of the successful trials and applications of collagen will make you far better informed if anyone asks you to explain the benefits!

ELASTEN CASE STUDY

The first study we will explore took place in 2019 with a sample size of 72 women, all of whom were 35 or older. This case study intended to determine the impact of Elasten, a drinkable form of collagen supplementation, on aging skin and overall skin health (Bolke et al., 2019). The basis of the case study relied on the fact that collagen is able to maintain skin structure and is known to, based on other studies, reverse the decrease of collagen synthesis due to age. Oral collagen supplements with specific collagen peptides showed signs of reversing the aging process due to the ability of the body to metabolize the peptides further and then release them into the bloodstream. Once these peptides are released, they form something called a "collagen biomatrix." Elasten, according to those who conducted the study, has a unique collagen complex with certain amino acid peptides that are more efficient at accomplishing the goals sought by those taking collagen supplement.

This study was conducted as a randomized, single-blind, placebo-controlled study. This means that the placebo and control groups were chosen entirely randomly, with no preferential treatment to who belonged to which group. The term "placebo

COLLAGEN IS LIFE | 109

controlled" means that participants in one group of the study were offered something that was not the collagen supplement, but were told it was. Placebo groups are vital in studies similar to this because they prove that people who were not given the substance being tested did not improve in the same ways that those taking the substance, in this case, Elasten, improved. The study being double-blind simply means that no one besides the person in charge of the study knew which group was the placebo or the control group, this includes any other researchers or assistants involved, and helps ensure that all data is unbiased. Participants, as I mentioned, included 72 women of ages 35 and up. The women involved in the study had to have considerably healthy skin. Women with skin diseases, other major diseases, heavy allergies, cancer, or with a history of drug use impacting the skin, were excluded, alongside women who were pregnant or breastfeeding, sunbathed recently, or used skin products containing active ingredients before the study began.

This study was conducted over the course of 12 weeks. After 12 weeks of taking either the placebo or the collagen supplement offered, subjects were then given a four week period without either substance before being examined. After this four week period, subjects who did take the collagen supplement were observed to see if the collagen treatment had sustained a four week period. The safety of the study was determined in various ways. Specifically, dermatological exams were conducted at all stages of the study to ensure that subjects were tolerating the substance well and without adverse effects. Adverse effects were monitored via self-reporting by all subjects throughout the study, and participants were asked again after the study to provide an evaluation as to whether or not they had suffered any adverse reactions from the product. This was in order to ensure that, when released or tested outside of a laboratory setting, the product would be safe.

At the end of the study, the results were analyzed and determined that the product was well tolerated. The results sustained the four week period fairly well, skin hydration was significantly improved by the group who took the collagen supplement, while the placebo group did not show similar results, skin elasticity improved significantly in the subjects, and skin roughness decreased dramatically. Improvements in skin density were also noticed. Due to the variety as well as the sustainability of the improvements that the supplement showed upon the skin, Elasten can be considered to be, based on this study, a very successful supplement.

So, why should you care about this particular case study? It is simple–after just 12 weeks of taking a collagen supplement consistently, even without any other lifestyle changes, participants in this study enjoyed significant improvements in the quality of their skin that were not just subjective. These results were objectively measured via criteria and tools, and sustained four weeks after the study at least. This means that even after the group stopped taking the supplement, for four weeks or more they enjoyed the same benefits with no decline. In other words, this supplement not only created significant improvements during the time period of being taken actively, but created such improvements that they did not disappear after the collagen supplement was no longer taken. Relative to you, this should indicate the sheer awesomeness that collagen has to offer. This study only focused on the skin as well, meaning positive impacts on nails, hair, organs, and joints weren't even recorded during this study. This case study goes to show that collagen really works, and is absolutely worth incorporating into your daily routine.

COLLAGEN & ANTIOXIDANTS

This next study observed the impacts of a collagen dietary supplement on improving various properties of the skin, such as texture (Genovese et al., 2017). The supplement provided in this study contained a blend of both collagen bioactive peptides and antioxidants. The background of this particular study states that, as a result of the aging process we all experience, skin suffers a loss of development or function in hyaluronic acid, collagen, and elastin (the material responsible for producing elastic in the various connective tissues throughout the body). As a result of these declines, the health and appearance of skin suffer with age.

The goal of this study was to observe the aesthetic and physical benefits of an oral collagen supplement composed of both collagen and antioxidants. This served to determine if the supplement was effective in counteracting the effects of the aging process on the skin. This study was double-blind, meaning that neither the participants nor the researcher knew which group was the control and which was the placebo. Double-blind studies are notoriously excellent at removing potential for bias or other issues with examining data. This study was also randomized and placebo-controlled, much like the last one. This one, however, studied 120 participants over the course of a 90-day period.

The sample subjects were split into two groups of 60 on a completely random basis. Each group was provided with one 50mL bottle of a substance daily; one group with the collagen and antioxidant blend and the other with the placebo liquid. Results of this study were measured based on skin elasticity and other objective, skin-related observations, and the participants engaged in self-guided questionnaires just like in the last study in order to self-report any effects.

The results of the study concluded that there was a significant improvement in skin texture and quality after consuming the collagen and antioxidant blend, whereas patients who took the placebo substance did not receive any of these benefits. Patients also provided a plethora of positive feedback via the questionnaires provided. This study concluded that this supplement is effective at protecting and improving the health of the skin. Much like the last study we discussed, this one goes to show that collagen can be incredibly beneficial for the health of the skin.

REVIEW OF VARIOUS STUDIES

Next, we will discuss an analysis of various collagen studies provided by Hsiuying Wang in 2021. In his work, Wang analyzes the "the effects of collagen treatment in different clinical studies including skin regeneration, bone defects, sarcopenia, wound healing, dental therapy, gastroesophageal reflux, osteoarthritis, and rheumatoid arthritis," as well as interpreted the possibility that someone with multiple of these diseases, including COVID-19, would be inherently collagen deficient (Wang, 2021). Overall, Wang determined that collagen-based treatment was highly effective at treating comorbid (meaning situations where someone has more than one of the aforementioned illnesses) diseases, improving overall health, and preventing further complications of each disease. Each of these diseases pertain specifically to something having to do with collagen stores. Let's take a closer look at some of Wang's findings to better understand the practical applications of both his work and the miracles collagen has to offer.

One case study mentioned by Wang discussed the impacts of marine collagen and its ability to maintain the health of the skin. In a study by Evans et al.– randomized, placebo-controlled, and single-blind–the effectiveness of marine collagen was observed. This studied hydrolyzed collagen on women between 45 and 60 years old. The results of the Evans et al. case study concluded that hydrolyzed marine collagen sourced from fish could improve and reverse the impacts of aging on skin. This means that the efficacy of marine collagen is significant enough to make marine-based collagen worth taking so long as the ingredients are specified. Wild-caught fish-based collagen supplements are far superior to ones that simply boast the label "marine collagen."

In another study, Asserin et al. studied how effective collagen peptide supplements were for hydrating the skin. The study lasted over the course of multiple weeks and the supplement provided showed astounding improvements in not just skin hydration, but collagen density improved and collagen damage decreased as well. What is particularly notable about this study is that the effects were weighed again 12 weeks after the study, meaning that participants had not taken collagen in 12 weeks post-study. Shockingly, the positive impacts of the collagen study lasted, and the study was able to conclude that collagen peptide supplements improve the effects of aging on the skin significantly. I am not saying to start a collagen supplement and then stop, but this study does prove that missing a day is not the end of the world and that the effects of a collagen supplement can be so powerful from just a few weeks of a consistent routine.

In a study by Tanaka et al., the impact of collagen on skin damage caused by sunlight radiation was observed. The study concluded that collagen is very effective at preventing sunlight-related skin damage, as throughout the process of the study the collagen supplement prevented skin dehydration and other negative effects sustained by the sun. Collagen studies have also provided significant evidence to support the effective nature of collagen in healing or minimizing the impact of various bone defects. Collagen-based medical intervention, for example, was able to strengthen the weakness of bones due to age.

Furthermore, collagen studies have determined that collagen can be incredibly useful with regard to dental therapy. For example, periodontitis is a severely prevalent dental disease that many adults have as a result of bacterial infection and other aspects of poor dental hygiene. This disease can cause teeth to fall out or need to be removed from the jaw if untreated. One study by Tizzoni and Tizzoni showed how a tooth could be preserved via periodontal regeneration surgery, which implemented collagen membranes as a part of a bone graft to improve bone degeneration. Collagen has been effective at improving symptoms of gingival recession, complications in tooth extraction surgeries, healing post-operation dental surgery wounds, and reconstructing dental implants. Regarding dental-related collagen affairs, only certain types of collagen were highly-effective, specifically bovine, equine, and human collagen.

Another set of studies has proven that collagen is effective in minimizing the harsh symptoms of gastroesophageal reflux, more commonly known as GERD. For someone with GERD, stomach acid will bubble up from the stomach and into the esophagus. It can cause a drastic decrease in quality of life, lead to throat cancer, etc. Studies managed to link type I and III collagens with GERD. Collagen treatment for GERD showed that 10 patients experienced significant improvement of GERD symptoms when injected with collagen in various problem sites. The collagen supplement used in this study acted as a bulking agent to prevent symptoms of GERD. This is not something that has been done widely or expansively, but it is really amazing to see all of the different ways in which collagen can be used to our benefit.

Another incredible and amazing way collagen can be utilized is for osteoarthritis. Osteoarthritis, also referred to as OA, is one of the most common joint diseases and causes for disability. OA occurs when joint cartilage and surrounding bone breaks down. It can be incredibly painful and debilitating. Collagen type II is the main form of collagen found in cartilage tissue impacted by OA. One trial surrounding collagen and OA took a sample of 39 patients who had been diagnosed with OA in the knee. 19 of these patients were, during the study, treated for their OA with solely acetaminophen, while the other 20 patients were treated with a combination of acetaminophen and a type II collagen supplement. The result of this particular study showed that the treatment mixed with collagen type II was far superior in improving OA symptoms in the participants. Collagen overall works very well for OA as one method to combine with others because it is incredibly safe and effective. If you are suffering from joint pain, collagen is a fantastic way to try to alleviate some of that suffering.

Similar to OA, rheumatoid arthritis (also known as RA) is an autoimmune and inflammatory disorder which primarily affects the joints. RA causes cartilage and bone to erode as a result of fibrovascular tissue invasion. Collagen type II administered orally via a supplement was beneficial to subjects with RA as well; there are many major studies that prove this. For example, one study analyzed 274 patients who were diagnosed with rheumatoid arthritis. This group was randomly placed into either a placebo group or another group which received varying dosages of a collagen type II supplement over the course of a 24-week period. Even with the lowest dose provided, patients showed signs of many positive effects as opposed to the placebo group who saw no improvements. This study utilized collagen derived from chicken breast, and vastly improved the symptoms patients with RA experienced.

Wang also reviewed a study involving the effects of collagen on COVID-19 in his work. COVID-19 is, from a scientific standpoint, a severe acute respiratory syndrome that has impacted nearly 200 million people

COLLAGEN IS LIFE | 119

worldwide. Undoubtedly, you or someone you know was, or still is, being impacted by the COVID-19 pandemic that ravaged our planet. What researchers discovered pertaining to collagen and the COVID-19 virus indicated that collagen treatment may be a valid protective agent that serves to protect the body and immune system from viruses. Furthermore, studies have indicated that COVID-19 resulted in a bodily tendency to break down or attack the body's own collagen stores. In turn, it seems promising that collagen would have the potential to treat COVID-19 and its related symptoms, along with other illnesses that could occur. While the research is still inconclusive because COVID-19 is still new in terms of medical history, the benefits of collagen allow collagen to be a useful nutritional supplement to reduce complications in sick individuals, including COVID-19 patients.

Wang's analysis of this set of case studies serves as incredible evidence for the powers of collagen to heal various ailments that the body could face for any reason. His work represents just a tiny fraction of the available case studies and research available on collagen, but all of them point to the same conclusion. I particularly enjoyed reading Wang's paper evaluating various collagen case studies because Wang does a phenomenal job at cross referencing in the evaluations offered, and this work is great for learning about scientific benefits of collagen more generally.

COLLAGEN GEL STUDIES

Another form of case study that has been extensively researched by those interested in the benefits of collagen supplementation includes collagen gel studies. Collagen gels have been used in many studies for many reasons by a wide variety of patients. A collagen gel is mostly water, consisting of only 1% collagen, but that 1% sure can work miracles (Dodla, 2008). The intended use of collagen gel is to benefit topical cell growth. Collagen gel is known to be able to escalate the rate of cell regrowth or regeneration, which means its positive impact on wounds has been extensively researched.

Collagen gel works in a few ways. One of the common ways it has been used is to fill vein grafts in order to allow nerves to repair at a much faster rate while also avoiding the potential of the vein to collapse. Studies in fact showed that vein grafts which employed collagen fillings experienced a significant amount of healing and growth compared to grafts without. This is because collagen gel is phenomenal at allowing nerves to sprout and grow. Collagen gels also use well hydrolyzed collagen, which can be absorbed more easily by the body since the peptides within hydrolyzed collagen weigh less than in other forms of collagen. The hyaluronic acid components of collagen gel have also allowed this product to be effective at preventing scarring. Allow me to walk you through a few case studies that show this amazing breadth of improvement that collagen gel can provide.

The first case study I will discuss was carried out by Maria Goddard, who studied a specific 74-year-old man–a nursing home resident (Goddard, 2021). The male being observed for this case had a history of, according to Goddard, "cerebral infarction, hemiplegia, hypertension, hyperlipidemia, urinary tract infection, pulmonary embolism and atrial fibrillation." On the first day of the study, the patient had a wound presenting 1.6 cm by 2 cm by 0.4 cm, which was classified as a stage four pressure ulcer. This patient sustained the injury just after he experienced a cerebral infarction with hemiplegia. In other words, this wound developed shortly after he sustained a stroke with partial paralysis of one side of the body.

The typical treatment for a wound of this degree was applied, yet the patient showed no improvement and was, therefore, intended to go for plastic surgery to heal the wound. However, after simply cleaning the wound with saline and then applying a hydrolyzed collagen powder and gauze, just five weeks later the wound was healed and the patient was discharged without any need for surgical intervention. The results of this study were particularly astounding, even to me as someone with extensive experience in collagen products. In 14 days, the size of the wound shrunk noticeably and tissue began covering the exposed fat and bone beneath the skin. On day 21, the wound was less than a centimeter on any side, and by day 35, the wound was considered completely healed. That is absolutely amazing progress for an injury that was anticipated to need plastic surgery!

Another study of collagen for wound healing was conducted by Sachin Chopra on a male in his early 50s (Chopra, n.d.). According to Chopra, this patient had a history of blood pressure issues, kidney disease, elevated body mass index, sleep apnea, asthma, MRSA, neuropathy, muscle weakness, and more, many of which illnesses are chronic for this patient. The patient entered care complaining of a chronic ulcer that had persisted for two years and remained about the same size throughout those years. The wound showed no sign of healing and the patient tried a variety of at-home remedies for his injury. This wound was 5.5 cm by 2 cm by 0.6 cm, and was fairly severe aesthetically and moderately concerning medically. Doctors diagnosed this wound to be a chronic venous stasis wound, which is caused by the inability of an extremity to allow blood to flow back to the heart. In this case of this specific patient, this issue affected his leg.

Similar to the last study, treatment was administered after a simple saline cleanse. A hydrolyzed collagen gel was applied to the wound daily and covered in breathable dressings, alongside ACE bandage wraps and recommended leg elevation. Within a week, the wound showed significant levels of improvement, and within three, it was considered completely healed with minimal aftercare recommendations necessary.

The third and final hydrolyzed collagen gel case study we will cover was conducted by Chopra once again, and was arguably more gruesome of a wound than the last two. This patient was a 63-year-old male with a medical history of colitis, diabetes, several amputation surgeries, muscle weakness, ulcers, and other ailments. A skin graft was conducted to close a chronically pervasive wound on his lower right leg, which reopened prior to the graft procedure. The patient then underwent something called a "revascularization" procedure, which is intended to improve blood circulation to the area in which the skin graft was conducted. Various treatments were applied to the rather large wound, and even after two months, no significant nor sustained improvement was modeled. This wound covered a surface of over 18 by 2 centimeters, far larger than the last two mentioned.

Once again, saline was used to cleanse the wound. Then the same hydrolyzed collagen gel used in the other studies was applied daily along with non-adhesive based dressing and bandages. Physical therapy, including leg elevation, was also employed. Within 14 amazing days, this wound was considered completely healed. Again, within 14 days, a wound treated for two months that resisted all treatment was cured with collagen gel.

It is important to keep in mind both the age and conditions of all of these patients. Despite being at a later stage in life and being afflicted by multiple severe, chronic diseases and illnesses, each of these three patients enjoyed an incredible improvement in the healing process of their wound as a result of the use of collagen gel. As such, if you have found yourself fighting a stubborn topical wound that you are sure is not infected, as was the case in all of these studies, a collagen gel might be perfect for you. Many wound creams and gels are available online and over the counter that contain collagen gel, the majority of which are pretty cheap. Keep in mind that these gels only work for topical wounds, not any of the internal nor broad skin health benefits of collagen. Overall, I definitely do recommend keeping a collagen gel on hand or in your first aid kit!

MUSCLE STRENGTH & SARCOPENIA CASE

In this next case study, we will explore the benefits of collagen on elderly men with sarcopenia. In case you are not already familiar with what sarcopenia is, let me explain: "Sarcopenia" is the term referring to the steady decline in skeletal muscle tissue as someone approaches old age. This might not sound as severe as it is, but sarcopenia is the leading cause of health decline and a loss of independence that comes with age. Sarcopenia is debilitating in a literal sense and devastating for any sufferers and loved ones who experience it. Fortunately, case studies involving sarcopenic patients and collagen have exhibited promising results from the use of collagen in improving this harrowing illness.

This specific study observed approximately 60 men over the age of 65 who were otherwise healthy and met criteria for the study, but showed signs of sarcopenia development when tested for their muscle strength and mass (Zdzieblik et al., 2015). This study involved putting these participants through a three month long resistance training, so only individuals who met all of those aspects were allowed to participate. Each subject underwent a comprehensive medical exam and then were split into two groups. One group received a collagen peptide supplement throughout the course of the study; the other received the placebo substance. The study was conducted based on randomization and was double-blind. For the duration of the course of the study, those who were part of the treatment group received 15 grams of collagen supplement a day, whereas the other group received a safe food additive called "silica." The supplement and placebo was delivered in the form of a powder mixed into water that they were told to drink within an hour of completing training. During the first hour post-exercise, participants cannot consume anything besides water.

53 of the subjects completed the study, with the outlying seven having missed training sessions. Muscle strength and mass along with other benefits were observed in both groups, though the results after the duration of the study concluded that the group who took the collagen peptide supplement experienced far more significant improvements compared to the placebo group. The study, therefore, concluded that collagen peptides were able to increase the benefits of working against sarcopenia in elderly patients. This is, as a matter of fact, excellent news, because it means that collagen is promising in allowing people who are aging to retain independence, mobility, and overall degrees of their quality of life. Collagen peptide supplementation

alongside exercise is, as proven by this study, a valuable way to improve muscle strength that is lost from sarcopenia.

MENOPAUSE & COLLAGEN

We have talked in depth about the benefits of collagen to specifically the aging male population, but that does not mean that collagen is without benefit for the aging female population. In fact, it is quite the opposite! This next case study observed the ability of collagen peptide supplementation to improve bone density and other bone-related health signs in postmenopausal women (König et al., 2018).

As a result of collagen testing on rodents, and throughout in vitro experimentation, scientists were alerted to the fact that collagen peptides had the ability to positively influence bone formation as well as the mineral density of bones, which then spurred on a further study. For the duration of a randomized, placebo-controlled and double-blind study, 131 women were investigated for shifts in bone mineral density of the neck and spine after a year-long period. Plasma levels and type I collagen were also observed in this study. All women were postmenopausal and experienced a significant decline in bone mineral density as a result of the aging process. Only 102 of the women completed the study, but the results were promising. According to the study, specific collagen peptides tested were able to significantly improve bone health in post-menopausal women, meaning that much of the bone loss and degradation faced as a result of menopause had been improved upon or negated altogether. This study just goes to show that there is some benefit of collagen for anyone to appreciate.

That is a lot of case studies validating the positive impacts of collagen supplements, and the ones above make up the tiniest percentage of studies indicating the same things: Collagen supplements are amazing for the skin, body, and your overall health. Collagen case studies have provided undeniable evidence supporting the power it holds. From just this small sample of case studies, we have indisputable evidence that collagen can aid with various illnesses, wound healing, and symptoms of aging that were once thought to be unhelpable.

At any age and with any health condition, there is a lot of positive news for those looking into collagen supplements of any form. Whether you are starting young or old, male or female, injured or well, collagen is, without a doubt, scientifically proven to benefit you in some way. Hopefully, you feel a lot more confident in the powers of collagen after reading the information on those studies. I know I did once I saw the vast amount of scientific support for collagen. Next, we are going to talk about how to actually weed out supplements to narrow down the one that works best for you.

7

HOW TO PICK THE RIGHT PRODUCT

Walking into the store and buying a collagen supplement for the first time can be a very daunting process–there are so many options, and at a glance, it can be hard to find the right product for you. There are a few important things to consider when picking out a collagen supplement that will make the process of purchasing your first one smooth sailing.

First things first, if you are using a store-bought collagen supplement to boost and protect your body's collagen, you should opt for a supplement that is made from all organic sources. From pills to powders, your collagen supplement should be as natural as can be. Your collagen should be sourced from cows fed on grass, seafood caught wild, or chickens that were raised free-range (MD & Michael, 2021). This helps ensure that your collagen supplement will be free of antibiotics, hormones, or GMO-based ingredients that can impact how well the collagen supplement works in your body. When searching for an all-natural collagen supplement, make sure you look out for how it is labeled. If the ingredient list contains the phrase "natural sources," then the brand is claiming that minimal amounts of processing, synthetic dyes or flavors, and preservatives were used. It might sound perfect to grab a supplement that says it is made with all natural sources, but I would advise against doing so without researching carefully. Compounds along the lines of antibiotics or hormones are not technically considered to be artificial ingredients, and therefore, a supplement claiming to be sourced naturally may be full of antibiotics. Instead, look for labels that say "all-natural" because this means that the brand is guaranteeing that the product is both free of dyes and flavorings as well as antibiotics and other compounds you will want to avoid.

Something else you will want to look for is collagen that says it is hydrolyzed. While all collagen is technically hydrolyzed, the products labeled as such are better because the amino acids that compose the collagen peptides are broken down further. This makes the collagen easier to digest, flavorless, and able to be mixed into any drink, hot or cold. Well-hydrolyzed collagen has been observed to be more effective in benefiting the body than collagen that has not undergone a thorough hydrolyzation process.

It is also a good idea to search for a collagen supplement with a diverse amino acid profile. Our body utilizes over a dozen different amino acids to function on a daily basis, and those amino acids are necessary for collagen growth as well. Finding the supplement available to you with the most diverse profile of amino acids is the best way to ensure that your collagen supplement will work best for you.

It is also my recommendation that you avoid collagen with sources labeled simply as "marine" collagen. Unless the marine collagen you find has specified the exact ingredients that make it up, it is better to avoid it. This is because marine collagen is a relatively varied and unregulated term–with marine collagen you could be getting anything, and not all sources of marine collagen are easily digested. For instance, shark and jellyfish collagen cannot be absorbed by the body as easily as collagen from fish is. Marine collagen also runs the risk of being exposed to certain marine allergens since the ingredients are not specified.

PRODUCT ANALYSIS: PROS AND CONS

Weighing the pros and cons of various products can be overwhelming, considering how many there are on the market. It requires a lot of rigorous research, comparison, note-taking, and can be a hassle generally. Discouraging, even. While I still encourage you to do your own research and understand what ingredients make up the exact product you are looking at, I have done a lot of the heavy lifting of research for you. I will give you the broad, overarching pros and cons of the most popular collagen supplement brands or products, and then all you have to do is verify the ingredients and that the product is best suited for your needs. Please note that I am not sponsored by or selling any of these products; I simply want to make sure you have access to some of the preliminary research you will need throughout the decision making process.

The first product that I will discuss is Youtheory Collagen with Vitamin C. This is a popular supplement that many people consider when searching for their first supplement. Youtheory is one of the cheapest, more budget-friendly options that I will list, which comes with its own set of benefits and drawbacks. Youtheory Collagen is NSF-certified, for starters (Link, 2022). Products that are NSF-certified undergo something called "third-party testing." During the process of third-party testing, an independent company with no stakes in the product or involvement in its creation tests the quality of the product. Generally speaking, NSF-certified and third-party tested products are ideal because they are backed by the word of an independent company that has no reason to try and make the product seem better than it is. NSF-certified products are generally a bit more trustworthy. I also mentioned that this product is on the cheaper end of the available options, making it a good choice for anyone on a strict budget. I do recommend paying for options that are a little more costly if they have a leverage beneficially, and therefore I think Youtheory is best for cost effectiveness only. This product has less collagen than other supplements on the market and comes in a tablet that is relatively big in size, causing customers to complain of it being hard to swallow. Overall, this product is great for anyone looking for a cheap, yet trustworthy, collagen supplement.

Another product that many people look into is Anthony's Hydrolyzed Marine Collagen Peptides. This product is a bit more expensive than the last but is still very cost effective as far as collagen supplements go. Despite the name containing the phrase "marine collagen," the brand states that their collagen is sourced from wild-caught fish, meaning that this is an incredibly natural supplement. This product is batch tested and gluten-free, although it is not third-party tested. The company also says that this product has no flavor, but some customers reported a slight fishy taste or smell. If this is something that would bother you immensely, this may not be the best supplement for you.

Further Food Collagen Peptides is another brand of collagen supplement that you might find in your research. They are also relatively cost effective considering the benefits. This brand is third party-tested, but not NSF-certified. Further Food Collagen Peptides only contain one ingredient–collagen sourced from grass fed cows. This product is incredibly natural and relatively effective, but it does contain a lower dose of collagen compared to some other supplements. Taste wise, some people reported a bad taste, however, if you are mixing the powder into a drink or food item that is strongly flavored, this might not be an issue. For those searching for a reliable, natural, and cost-friendly option for a collagen powder, this may be a product worth looking into further.

Sports Research Collagen Peptides Powder is the last of the more affordable options I will list. This option is affordable as well as certified keto and paleo; those who follow either of these diets should absolutely research this product further if they are struggling to find a suitable product. This product is also third-party tested as well as certified, setting it apart as more reliable of a supplement than some other options. The ingredients list is short, which is definitely a good thing when looking for any supplement. A short ingredients list means that the product is more likely to be free of additives, flavors, preservatives, or other unnatural substances that you do not want your supplement to have. On the negative side, people who have used this product also thought that there were some negative flavors associated with it. Customers also experienced a bit of clumping when trying to mix the product into cold liquids, which can be less than desirable if you plan to use your protein powder for colder drinks. Overall, I had suggested this product for people mixing their collagen powder into hot drinks or foods and who do not care about the taste of the product.

Care/of Collagen is one of the more expensive products that people tend to love. The major drawback of this product is that you have to have a subscription to buy the product, meaning overall this product can run you a decent bit of cash. Even still, there are tons of benefits to enjoy if you opt to spend the money on this product. For starters, Care/of Collagen produces multiple flavors of collagen powder to choose from, which is something a lot of brands with similar levels of quality do not offer. This brand is also third-party tested, and it is easy to blend too. You are not likely to experience any clumps or grainy textures with this powder. Care/of Collagen powder is also very well hydrolyzed, so the body will be able to absorb this supplement far better than some other supplements that are not quite as hydrolyzed. If you are interested in collagen supplements long term and have a good amount of money to dedicate to the venture, research Care/of Collagen and see if their products are a good fit for you and your needs.

Vital Proteins Collagen Peptides is another potential option for those seeking a good collagen powder. This brand is also third-party tested, and you can purchase their powder in a tub just like with the majority of other brands, or in a stick form for convenience. I mentioned in another chapter how helpful vitamin C and hyaluronic acid are to the maintenance and development of collagen. One of the reasons that this product is so awesome is that it contains a good amount of both vitamin C and hyaluronic acid, allowing the product to be just a notch above some of the rest. The downside of this product is that it can be very expensive and the flavor is rather bad.

Vital Proteins sells another highly recommended product called Vital Proteins Beauty Collagen. It is third-party tested and available in multiple flavors, which is a major selling point if you are using it to make yourself a flavorful beverage infused with collagen. This product contains hyaluronic acid just like the Vital Proteins Collagen Peptides product does, but instead of vitamin C, this one contains probiotics. The major drawbacks of this particular product include being more expensive than competitors' products and dissolving poorly in cold liquids.

Another option for collagen supplements that many people are interested in is Garden of Life Grass Fed Collagen Beauty. As with many of the other products listed, complaints exist solely within the realm of price and taste. Otherwise, this seems to be a stellar product with many benefits and reasons to give it a chance. This product is third-party tested, NSF-certified, and fits an array of dietary needs. Namely, this supplement is gluten-free as well as keto and paleo-friendly. As opposed to many other brands, this one contains a myriad of additional supplements to boost the growth and protection of your collagen, hair, skin, and nails. Garden of Life contains vitamin C, probiotics, biotin, and silica, all of which are desirable in a supplement of this variety. This is absolutely one of the better options on the list if price is not an issue for you.

Thorne Collagen Plus is another good option. Produced in a third-party certified lab, this collagen supplement is specifically intended to benefit your hair and skin. It is flavored naturally and has no added sugars, although it is a bit pricier than similar products. One major con that could be a concern is that while the product was produced in a third-party certified facility, the product itself is not third-party tested. This means it is ultimately up to you how much you trust the product.

Klean Collagen+C is a little bit different from some of the other products here, because not only is it NSF third-party certified, but this supplement is specifically certified for athletic use. It contains a good amount of vitamin C per serving, is well hydrolyzed to result in flawless absorption, and has a high amount of collagen in each serving. It is a pricier option with a strong flavor, but nonetheless, one that people with active lifestyles may find best suited for their needs.

The final product on this list is HUM Nutrition Collagen Love. This is a powder also available in capsule form, and it is third-party tested. The product is composed of a blend of herbal ingredients alongside collagen in order to benefit the skin specifically. Unfortunately, this product is relatively expensive while simultaneously containing a lower dose of

COLLAGEN IS LIFE | 141

collagen than the majority of other products of the same price.

Having a strong basic background on some of the majority of other popular collagen supplements people look into is a great way to start narrowing down your options for your first supplement. If one of the above products sounds as if it is perfect for what you are looking for, make sure to research it a bit more. Look into the doses, ingredients, prices, and more to determine if that is the right supplement for you.

SUPPLEMENTS ON A BUDGET

As unfortunate as it is, more and more people nowadays are faced with the unfortunate circumstance of being strapped for cash. Collagen supplements are admittedly one of the more pricier things you can end up spending money on in the name of health. Because of this, I have compiled a couple of cheaper collagen supplement options that are more cost effective than the ones above. Though I do have to stress that I recommend paying for a more expensive supplement if you can. With the proper research and consideration, you will be able to avoid any gimmicky products or ones that flat out do not work with ease. For cheaper supplements, you do get what you pay for; namely, a cheaper collagen supplement is more likely to contain lower levels of collagen and result in less of the positive effects that you are looking for with a supplement.

Vital Proteins, one of my favorite and mostly highly recommended brands, can be expensive, but they do carry cheaper options for single-use collagen available at drug stores. Besides that, I can't really say that I would recommend a specific brand, but I do recommend checking the store brands and cheaper brands available in your store the right way. As I have mentioned before, checking the ingredients list is going to be your best bet for ensuring that the collagen supplement you select will work. You will want to pick a supplement that is both specific and low on ingredients, because the less ingredients listed the more pure the collagen usually is.

Outside of budget-friendly collagen supplements, I recommend a multivitamin and a vitamin C supplement. These are usually the cheapest options for nutritional supplements available, and as you know from the duration of this book, both are fantastic for improving your collagen in a variety of ways. Even if you do not have the money to spend on fancy, expensive supplements, through your diet, exercise, and other supplements, you can still appreciate all of the same benefits collagen has to offer.

In this chapter, you learned about the various things to look for and avoid in a collagen supplement. We covered various specific options for supplements as well as the pros and cons of each. In this next and final chapter, I will cover some of my more personalized recommendations based on the supplements I have taken and their results.

8

MY RECOMMENDATIONS

Alright, so why did I go through the process of listing all of those previous products only to have a whole chapter on my personal recommendations? Personally, I think the research shows that all of the products I listed off in the last chapter are all potentially great options for collagen supplements. Customers seem overwhelmingly happy with the results, and scientifically, the products check out. However, not all of those products are ones I have taken myself. Here, I want to highlight a couple of products that I have personally taken for years at a time along with the benefits they provided for me.

All of the supplements I listed before are pretty solid options; I can say that if I were starting out, I would feel confident in taking any one of those options. None of them are particularly bad for you in any way, but on my personal journey I started a bit differently. I mentioned the Vital Proteins brand already. That is the brand I started with and the brand I recommend that you start with as well. I suggest taking the Vital Proteins basic collagen option and see if you like it personally. That is the supplement I began with and took for over a year. I purchased the brand from Costco and do not at all regret my decision. The results were noticeable.

Vital Proteins has several popular options including the original and beauty options, so there is sure to be a version of the product that will work best for your collagen-related goals. This product is worth the price, but the price is in fact pretty high. I recommend checking the prices at Costco if you live near one or purchasing a subscription—this can make the high cost of the product go down dramatically. For more athletic individuals, I definitely recommend the sports research powder brand.

Nowadays, taking collagen supplements in powder form has become incredibly inconvenient for me personally. I travel a lot for work, which means it is not at all times easy to mix a powder into a food or drink item. Because of this, I have since switched to pill and capsule forms of collagen in order to take them conveniently and all at once. My go to supplement now is the

YouTheory pill form of collagen supplement, and I take six of the capsules during lunch. I have been taking these supplements for over a year now, and the dosage is a bit smaller than when I was taking Vital Proteins. You can buy YouTheory supplements from Amazon or directly through their website, though I do recommend starting off with a collagen powder first.

I have tons of other recommendations for collagen supplements as well–years of devotion to research and my health have granted me the ability to speak on so many other products. One of the other products that I really suggest is Ancient Nutrition. While on the more expensive side, Ancient Nutrition is a premium brand that uses high quality ingredients and offers a fantastic line of supplements. If you try Vital Proteins and find that it is not for you, this should be your next go to product.

FURTHER RESEARCH

If, after reading this book, you feel inspired to do more research on collagen and anything else I have mentioned, first of all, I am elated for you. Your spurred interest in collagen, collagen dieting, the benefits of collagen, and how to improve your life with collagen is going to be one of the best things to happen to you. Second, I am going to offer you some essential advice for the rest of your research process–advice that has been instrumental in guiding me through my research that I want to share with you too.

First, it is important to compare a variety of sources on things you are not sure about. If one source says something about collagen, but five others contradict it, that first source is likely not as reliable. Finding sources that support each other and back each other up with a combination of scientific evidence and experience are going to be your best bet regarding superior and credible sources on collagen (or anything, really). Second, you are going to want to check the currency of any source you plan to use because of the fact that science is constantly evolving. A resource on collagen from 1970 is not going to be as reliable or credible as a source from 2017 is, for example. Finally, I would recommend looking into the author of any source you plan to trust, especially regarding collagen and other things that you plan to put into your body. If someone is a doctor and studies collagen as a specialty, they are almost certainly more reliable than someone selling you a product with no reviews online from a Facebook ad.

VIDEO RECOMMENDATIONS

Additionally, for anyone interested in further research relating to collagen, products, or anything related, or for anyone who just wants to watch some video analysis of collagen and its associated factors, I have some videos and YouTube channels I personally favor and suggest checking out. The reason I recommend checking out some video sources regarding collagen as you continue learning is that I wholeheartedly believe in approaching health in a way that combines knowledge and experience. This book has focused substantially on scientific ways to improve and preserve your collagen levels alongside my personal experience, and that is, in my opinion, the best way to go about a health change. Combining knowledge from professionals and experience from those who have engaged in a habit for years is a guaranteed way to get the most out of your research.

The first video I would recommend checking out is SimplyDivineCurls' "4 YEAR UPDATE" video. She has been taking collagen peptides for four years, and in this video she provides in depth updates on the benefits that her collagen supplement routine has provided for her hair. In the description of her video, she also recommends a ton of awesome products that she enjoys and I support as well due to my experience with them. If you are looking for someone to talk about the benefits of collagen on maintaining healthy and resilient hair, this is definitely the channel you will want to check out. Plus, collagen benefits toward hair also tend to benefit the skin and nails as well, so overall she is a very good content creator to give some love if you feel like you want more information on the benefits of collagen supplements, specifically collagen powder, toward the hair, skin, and nails.

The next video I would suggest is the "Vital Proteins Collagen Peptides | Results" video posted on Keto with JT's channel. At the time of posting this specific video, he was six months into his journey and he provides many valuable tips and important feedback regarding various collagen powder supplements. He also has multiple playlists on his channel that include videos he has made for different aspects of collagen related benefits. So many different facets of collagen information are covered on JT's channel, and all of his information is as true as can be, earning him a spot on my list of favorite collagen-related YouTubers. This is overall one of my favorite channels to visit when I am searching for something collagen-related to watch on YouTube.

The final video I will recommend is "Do Collagen Supplements Work?!" from the channel of The Budget Dermatologist. Her video is incredibly informative regarding the benefits of collagen, and her video is engaging with a lot of credible information. She goes over various aspects of collagen supplementation in a way that is a great brief for anyone new to learning about the benefits of collagen. Her channel does focus mostly on skincare given its namesake, so if you are seeking skincare related advice, her channel is a must have resource.

In this chapter, you learned about my specific and personal recommendations for collagen supplements and some valuable tips for collagen research moving forward as well. Overall, I guarantee you cannot go wrong testing out anything I mentioned in this chapter or the previous one so long as you follow the safety guidelines and are sure to avoid any potential negative side effects.

CONCLUSION

I hope you feel as if you have learned a lot of valuable information that you can apply towards the improvement of your life. In this book, you learned what collagen does for the body, the different types of collagen, how the body loses collagen, and how to prevent that loss. You have learned valuable tools for how to feel your body, you can now appropriately select a supplement for yourself and your needs, and you know the various ways in which incorporating a collagen supplement into your life can benefit you. From scientific evidence to my personal experience, you have gained so many tools to use moving forward, and I hope you feel confident in every single one of them. Now that you have all of this vital information, you are ready to begin a new chapter of your life—one where you look and feel as healthy as can be.

Collagen supplements are, in my opinion, one of the best things you can do for yourself. Soon your hair, skin, nails, bones, and joints will be flourishing just how they did years ago. Take what you have learned and get out there; pick a supplement you think you will like and start reaping the benefits. Remember, a combined approach of all of the different methods in this book—specifically supplementation, exercise, diet, and lifestyle changes—is going to allow you to see the most significant and long-lasting benefits from including collagen into your life. Now, you should have all the tools you need to feel confident in using collagen for your own benefit as well as encouraging others to do the same.

And finally, I appreciate you trusting me to take you on this journey. If you found the tips and information in this book valuable, consider leaving a review to allow others to find this book too. That way, we can all contribute to ensuring that this valuable information is not ignored; everyone can be the happy, healthy, vibrant version of themselves that they deserve to be, no matter what. I wish you luck on your collagen journey, and thank you for sticking with me for the ride!

REFERENCES

5 Research Studies That Show That Collagen Protein Should Be a Part of Your Sports Injury Treatment. (n.d.). Frog Fuel Collagen Protein. Retrieved February 12, 2023, from https://frogfuel.com/blogs/news/5-reasons-collagen-protein-injury-recovery

Bolke, L., Schlippe, G., Gerß, J., & Voss, W. (2019). A Collagen Supplement Improves Skin Hydration, Elasticity, Roughness, and Density: Results of a Randomized, Placebo-Controlled, Blind Study. Nutrients, 11(10), 2494. https://doi.org/10.3390/nu11102494

Choi, F. D., Sung, C. T., Juhasz, M. L. W., & Mesinkovsk, N. A. (2019). Oral Collagen Supplementation: A Systematic Review of Dermatological Applications. Journal of Drugs in Dermatology: JDD, 18(1), 9–16. https://pubmed.ncbi.nlm.nih.gov/30681787/

Chopra, S. (n.d.). CASE STUDY CHRONIC VENOUS STASIS WOUND. Retrieved February 21, 2023, from https://sanaramedtech.com/wp-content/uploads/2021/04/FINAL-Chopra-Venous-Stasis-Cas-Study-4.7.2021.pdf

Collagen: What it is, Types, Function & Benefits. (2022, May 23). Cleveland Clinic. https://my.clevelandclinic.org/health/articles/23089-collagen

Davis, C. (2022). Collagen Diet: Collagen-Rich Foods for Healthy Joints, Skin & Hair. MedicineNet. https://www.medicinenet.com/collagen_diet/article.htm

Dodla. (2008). Collagen Gel - an overview | ScienceDirect Topics. Www.sciencedirect.com. https://www.sciencedirect.com/topics/neuroscience/collagen-gel

Further Food. (2017, January 4). 4 Benefits of Collagen for Weight Loss. Further Food. https://www.furtherfood.com/collagen-for-weight-loss/

Genovese, L., Corbo, A., & Sibilla, S. (2017). An Insight into the

Changes in Skin Texture and Properties following Dietary Intervention with a Nutricosmeceutical Containing a Blend of Collagen Bioactive Peptides and Antioxidants. Skin Pharmacology and Physiology, 30(3), 146–158. https://doi.org/10.1159/000464470

Goddard, M. (2021). CASE STUDY STAGE IV PRESSURE ULCER. https://sanaramedtech.com/wp-content/uploads/2021/04/FINAL-Goddard-Stage-IV-Case-Study-4.7.2021.pdf

Is Collagen Good for Gut Health? (n.d.). Indigo Collagen. https://www.indigocollagen.com/blogs/indigo-blog/is-collagen-good-for-gut-health

König, D., Oesser, S., Scharla, S., Zdzieblik, D., & Gollhofer, A. (2018). Specific Collagen Peptides Improve Bone Mineral Density and Bone Markers in Postmenopausal Women—A Randomized Controlled Study. Nutrients, 10(1), 97. https://doi.org/10.3390/nu10010097

León-López, A., Morales-Peñaloza, A., Martínez-Juárez, V. M., Vargas-Torres, A., Zeugolis, D. I., & Aguirre-Álvarez, G. (2019). Hydrolyzed Collagen—Sources and Applications. Molecules, 24(22), 4031. https://doi.org/10.3390/molecules24224031

Link, R. (2022, April 22). The 11 Best Collagen Supplements for Better Skin. Healthline. https://www.healthline.com/nutrition/best-collagen-for-skin#comparison

Lisa Turner. (2022, January 31). The Heart-Boosting Benefits Of Collagen You May Not Be Aware Of. Better Nutrition. https://www.betternutrition.com/conditions-and-wellness/heart-health/heal-your-heart-with-collagen/

Llamas, M. (2022). Types of Collagen | There are 5 Common Types of Collagen. Drugwatch.com. https://www.drugwatch.com/health/collagen/types/

Marengo, K. (2019). 13 Foods That Boost Your Body's Natural Collagen Production. Healthline. https://www.healthline.com/health/beauty-skin-care/collagen-food-boost#berries

MD, A. M., & Michael. (2021, September 13). What To Look For In Collagen Powder. Amy Myers MD. https://www.amymyersmd.

com/article/collagen-powder-sources/
#Heres_What_To_Look_For_In_Collagen_Powder

Miller, K. (2020, March 10). Yes, The Sun Zaps Collagen From Your Body + 5 Other Reasons It Declines. Mindbodygreen. https://www. mindbodygreen.com/articles/the-reasons-collagen-declines-how-to-support-it-naturally

Muscleblaze. (2019). Muscleblaze. https://www.muscleblaze.com/arti cles/Supplements/top-6-reasons-why-collagen-is-a-gift-for-weight-training-individuals/8883

Reisdorf, A. (2019, March 8). Here's What You Need to Know About Vegan Collagen. Healthline; Healthline Media. https://www.health line.com/health/food-nutrition/vegan-collagen#creating-vegan-collagen

Team, T. C. E. (2019, January 17). 6 Herbs To Boost Collagen: Everything You Need To Know. The Chalkboard. https://thechalk boardmag.com/6-herbs-that-boost-collagen-adriana-ayales/

The Benefits Of Collagen For Hair, Skin & Nails. (2020, May 26). Rite-Flex. https://www.riteflexhealth.com/the-benefits-of-collagen-for-hair-skin-nails/

Van de Walle, G. (2021, December 21). Health Benefits of Collagen: Pros, Cons, and More. Healthline. https://www.healthline.com/nutrition/collagen-benefits#benefits

Wang, H. (2021). A Review of the Effects of Collagen Treatment in Clinical Studies. Polymers, 13(22), 3868. https://doi.org/10.3390/polym13223868

Zdzieblik, D., Oesser, S., Baumstark, M. W., Gollhofer, A., & König, D. (2015). Collagen peptide supplementation in combination with resistance training improves body composition and increases muscle strength in elderly sarcopenic men: a randomised controlled trial. British Journal of Nutrition, 114(8), 1237–1245. https://doi.org/10.1017/s0007114515002810